Praise for

You Won't Believe It's Vegan!

"*You Won't Believe It's Vegan!* really lives up to its title. Its wide variety of scrumptious recipes coupled with easy-to-follow directions will please vegans and non-vegans alike."

—Lois Dieterly, author of *Sinfully Vegan*

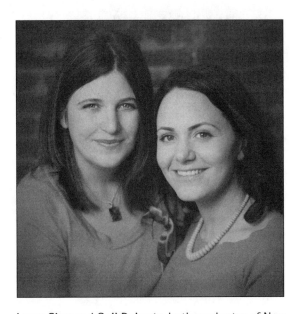

Lacey Sher and **Gail Doherty**, both graduates of New York City's Natural Gourmet Institute, in 1999 opened Down to Earth, New Jersey's first organic vegan restaurant, which they ran for seven years, until 2006. Lacey Sher owns a catering company and is opening a new organic, sustainable, vegetarian restaurant. She lives in Oakland, California, with her husband. Gail Doherty is a specialty vegan chef designing cuisine for America's second largest natural supermarket, in addition to providing restaurant consulting focused on natural foods and the importance of local agriculture. She lives in Asheville, North Carolina, with her husband and daughter.

You Won't
Believe It's
Vegan!

You Won't Believe It's Vegan!

200 Recipes for Simple and Delicious Animal-Free Cuisine

LACEY SHER and GAIL DOHERTY

Da Capo
LIFE
LONG

A Member of the Perseus Books Group

Many of the designations used by manufacturers and sellers to distinguish their products are claimed as trademarks. Where those designations appear in this book and Da Capo Press was aware of a trademark claim, the designations have been printed in initial capital letters.

Copyright © 2008 by Lacey Sher and Gail Doherty

Originally published as *Down to Earth Cookbook* by Pollinator Press in the United States, Copyright © 2006 by Lacey Sher and Gail Doherty.
All photographs by Bob McKay and Elisabeth Koch McKay
www.mckayimaging.com

All rights reserved. No part of this publication may be reproduced, stored in a retrieval system, or transmitted, in any form or by any means, electronic, mechanical, photocopying, recording, or otherwise, without the prior written permission of the publisher. Printed in the United States of America.

Designed by Pauline Brown.
Set in 11 point Granjon by the Perseus Books Group

Library of Congress Cataloging-in-Publication Data

Sher, Lacey, 1974–
    You won't believe it's vegan! : 200 recipes for simple and delicious animal-free cuisine / Lacey Sher and Gail Doherty. — 1st Da Capo Press ed.
        p.   cm.
    Includes bibliographical references and index.
    ISBN-13: 978-1-60094-070-5 (alk. paper)
    ISBN-10: 1-60094-070-6 (alk. paper)
    1. Vegan cookery. I. Doherty, Gail, 1969- II. Title.
    TX837.S462886 2008
    641.5'636—dc22
                        2007046820

First Da Capo Press edition 2008

Published by Da Capo Press
A Member of the Perseus Books Group
www.dacapopress.com

NOTE: The information in this book is true and complete to the best of our knowledge. This book is intended only as an informative guide for those wishing to know more about health issues. In no way is this book intended to replace, countermand, or conflict with the advice given to you by your own physician. The ultimate decision concerning care should be made between you and your doctor. We strongly recommend you follow his or her advice. Information in this book is general and is offered with no guarantees on the part of the authors of Da Capo Press. The authors and publisher disclaim all liability in connection with the use of this book. The names and identifying details of people associated with events described in this book have been changed. Any similarity to actual persons is coincidental.

Da Capo Press books are available at special discounts for bulk purchases in the United States by corporations, institutions, and other organizations. For more information, please contact the Special Markets Department at the Perseus Books Group, 2300 Chestnut Street, Suite 200, Philadelphia, PA 19103, or call (800) 810-4145, extension 5000, or e-mail special.markets@perseusbooks.com.

3 4 5 6 7 8 9

Contents

Contents

Sandwiches and Wraps 95

Appetizers 109

Contents

Kids' Food   193

Introduction

When we opened Down to Earth, our organic, vegan, whole-foods restaurant in Red Bank, New Jersey, our objective was to create a place that would serve the world as well as the vegan community, a place where vegan diners could come regularly but to which they would also bring their families and friends regardless the food's being vegan. For a long time, vegan food had a reputation for being bland and boring, and we were out to disprove that. In sharing the food that we ourselves enjoyed, we were delighted that nonvegetarians showed up and loved what they ate: delicious, high-quality food prepared well. These recipes you'll find here, born out of that desire, were some of the favorites at Down to Earth.

While one of our goals is to create delicious, flavorful world cuisine that's so tasty you won't miss the animal products, we also emphasize eating organic, whole foods. Even though "organic," "sustainable," and even "local" have become buzzwords, commercially grown and produced products predominate in the market, and so we believe it is still important to pay attention to where your ingredients come from. When you buy organic, you are choosing food that's grown without the use of synthetic chemicals, additives, fertilizers, or pesticides. You are also supporting a way of farming that is not subsidized by the government. This means that organic farmers often pay into the system as taxpayers and with agricultural fees, but they seldom or never receive the funding that mainstream corporate farmers get. Buying organic means that the money you spend is helping to support the organic farmers. Buying from your local farmers' market or directly from a local farmer is an even more proactive way to help support an age-old, healthier way of producing food. By using fresh, flavorful, naturally grown produce, spices, oils, nuts, and legumes, you can help perpetuate a tradition that goes back to the original chefs of all cultures, who were 100 percent organic.

Of course, chemicals used in the growing of food aren't the only problem. The use of chemicals to make and process food is a major industry. New advances in food science technology, like factory automation and the refining of grains, has made possible products with long shelf lives and high profits. Just in the last few decades, frozen, freeze-dried, instant, and artificial foods have become the norm. Modern society has embraced these foods, trading its health for the allure of the quick and easy meal. The recipes in this book help move you back to a more healthful way of eating by using whole foods, such as unadulterated grains, beans, fruits, and vegetables. Not only are these foods better for you, they simply taste better. Our recipes are designed to maximize flavor, elevating vegan cuisine to new heights.

As vegans, it is also important to both of us to prepare food that is kind to animals. There is a profound connection between raising and slaughtering animals for meat and growing and cultivating crops with petrochemicals, artificial hormones, and pesticides that affect human hormones. Our advocacy of using fresh, local, animal-free ingredients in our recipes gives you the opportunity to dine without supporting factory farming and agribusiness.

Of course, the mere mention of "vegan" or "vegetarian" will almost always spark a debate. It is easy to get defensive about eating animals—on both sides of the argument. Religion, history, educated and noneducated opinion, and misinformation all complicate the issue. Unfortunately, most people automatically assume that being a vegan means believing that all nonvegans are bad people. For the same reasons that organic, whole foods are better for you and the Earth, so is choosing vegan food. Modern-day agriculture's dependence on higher yields accelerates topsoil erosion on our farmlands, rendering land less productive for crop cultivation and forcing the conversion of wilderness to grazing and farmlands. Animal waste from massive feedlots and factory farms is a leading cause of pollution in our groundwater and rivers. The United Nations Food and Agriculture Organization has linked animal agriculture to a number of other environmental problems, including the contamination of aquatic ecosystems, soil, and drinking water by manure, pesticides, and fertilizers; acid rain from ammonia emissions; greenhouse gas production; and depletion of precious water aquifers. With regard to human health, the overconsumption of animal products has contributed to rampant heart disease, soaring cholesterol levels, all types of cancers, obesity, diabetes, hypertension, and kidney stones, just to name a few major health concerns. Add to that the use of antibiotics, drugs, and hormones on severely overcrowded, overstressed animals, and you can see why we support vegan ideals.

Ultimately, our philosophy about food stems from our deep love for the Earth and animals that share it with us. When we eat food, we are filled with appreciation for the wonderful variety and abundance that surround us. It is our hope and belief that by choosing an animal-free diet, we are not contributing any unnecessary suffering in animals' lives. We also look at veganism as a way of lessening the huge impact that meat production places on the Earth's vital resources. To us, the most important ingredient in our food is love—our love for the Earth and its bounty and all of its creatures.

Whether you are new to vegan cuisine or have been preparing animal-free meals for years, there's something for everyone here. From vegan versions of classic meat-filled entrées to a section devoted to kid-friendly food, from our signature desserts and baked goods to an assortment of live food dishes that serve as a great introduction to raw cuisine, these recipes are easy to make, satisfying, and great additions to any diet. Simply put, this is food that's good for you, animals, and the planet.

With our restaurant, we had set out to open many minds and palates to a new, fresh way of eating, no matter what a person's diet choices were. We challenged ourselves daily so that when diners sat down at our tables, they would have their horizons expanded and would know, firsthand, that vegan cuisine is about much more than salad. In sharing these recipes, we hope that you enjoy making, eating, and sharing these dishes as much as we enjoyed creating them.

—Lacey Sher & Gail Doherty

Basic Kitchen Equipment

When you're shopping for kitchen equipment, there are many items to choose from. Here are some handy basic tools that we use all the time, and some nonessential but great-to-have others that we recommend.

THE ESSENTIALS

A variety of mixing bowls—Our first choice would be bowls made of stainless steel or glass.

A sharp knife—A good knife is a knife with which you feel comfortable cutting. There are many sizes, shapes, and weights. Most home and kitchen stores offer a good selection of professional-grade knives. A paring knife, a serrated bread knife, and a 6- to 8-inch chef's knife will see you through nearly any prep work. A heavy cleaver is useful for cutting through hard winter squashes or cracking open young coconuts. We recommend a high-carbon stainless-steel blade that is forged, not stamped, and has a full tang (which means the metal that forms the blade extends all the way to the end of the handle).

A good cutting board—This is a must-have! We favor one with a heavier weight. A wooden cutting board is our preference, but if you live in a household where the cutting board may be used for meat or poultry as well, a nonporous composite material would be best, or have one dedicated to only meats, fish, and poultry, and another for other foods. To keep your cutting board from slipping around, lay a damp towel down underneath the board.

Pots and pans—We like stainless steel with an aluminum core. Stainless steel is nonreactive and doesn't change the flavor of the food. Good pots and pans will last you a lifetime and are worth investing in. A good assortment to have: 2-quart and 4-quart saucepans, a 5- to 6-quart Dutch oven, a smaller skillet, and a larger sauté pan. One nonstick skillet is useful to have for delicate foods such as crepes. One large (8-quart) stockpot will be needed for soups, sauces, and stocks.

Measuring spoons—It is very important to get sturdy measuring spoons. Measuring spoons come in sets, with sizes ranging from ⅛ teaspoon to 1 tablespoon. When measuring dry ingredients such as baking soda and baking powder, be sure to level off the top with a knife, for accuracy.

Measuring cups—There are two types of measuring cups, one for dry ingredients and one for wet.

> **Dry measuring cups,** which are calibrated for dry ingredients only, typically have straight sides and come in sets ranging from ⅛ cup to 1 cup. When using, always level off the dry ingredients with a knife, for accuracy.

> **Glass or clear plastic measuring cups** are transparent and have graduated lines on the sides for measuring liquid ingredients. Using dry cups for liquid ingredients may not produce desired effects, especially in baking. A 1-cup, 2-cup, and 4-cup set would be ideal.

Whisk—This simple tool is used for mixing dressings, making smooth batters, and whipping air into mixtures.

Wooden spoon—A wooden spoon is a good tool for stirring without damaging the pan or reacting with food. Always make sure to wash it well after using it and to it let air-dry completely before putting it away.

Spatulas—Purchase a few in various materials:
You want at least one big, wide, flat **metal spatula** for turning pancakes and lifting cookies off of the baking sheet without breaking them.

Rubber or silicone spatulas can be used with nonstick cookware and work great for scraping down the sides of the blender or food processor when you're trying to get all of the finished product out of your work bowl.

Offset spatulas look slightly bent and can be used for applying frostings to cakes and leveling the tops of creamy batters and cheesecakes.

Electrical Appliances—A blender and food processor are two items that are a little pricier but really worth it. If taken care of, they can last you a very long time.

Blender (or immersion blender)—You can get a wonderful blender for a reasonable price. The more power the blender has, the better. Blenders are great for pureeing soups, sauces, smoothies, and dressings. The handheld immersion blender is ideal for small quantities and for pureeing soups in the pot without having to transfer hot soup in batches to a standing blender.

Food processor—Shredding and slicing blades are very useful for cutting a large quantity of vegetables; the metal S blade is used in many ways, from chopping nuts to blending pâtés.

Kitchen timer—In cooking, sometimes timing is everything, and it's easy to lose track of time in a busy kitchen. Digital timers that can time three different processes are particularly useful.

Baking sheets—You'll need at least two medium-size sturdy baking sheets. We use 12 by 18-inch aluminum half-sheet pans from a restaurant supply house, but any noninsulated baking sheet will do.

Baking pans—Of glass or aluminum, an 8-inch square and a 9 by 13-inch baking pan will cover you through everything from lasagne to brownies.

Baking parchment—Parchment keeps food from contacting with the baking pan, so it won't stick. It also makes cleanup a breeze.

Cake pans—In addition to the above pans, you'll need two 9-inch straight-sided cake pans and a 9- to 10-inch springform pan if you wish to be a baker.

Cooling racks—These are essential for cooling down baked items. We recommend that you have at least two on hand.

NONESSENTIAL
BUT NICE TO HAVE

Pie plate—A 9-inch glass or ceramic pie plate is necessary for the pies and quiches in this cookbook. A tart pan with a removable bottom is also nice to have, but not necessary.

Salad spinner—If you want to dry salad greens or herbs, a salad spinner is very helpful. You can get by without one, but they work very well. Drying helps keep greens and herbs fresher longer.

Juicer—In the past, we have used a centrifugal juicer, which grinds the vegetables and fruit and forces the juice through a strainer. For a couple of recipes, we call for a Champion brand, or masticating, juicer, which chews up the veggies and fruit and extracts the juice by forcing the pulp through rotating gears.

Dehydrator—This is particularly useful if you are a raw foodist. It's great for making such raw food items as crackers and crusts, as well as dehydrating fruit and nuts.

Pantry

A word about some basics, discussed in more detail beginning on page 10. In general, read the fine print of labels carefully to be sure the products you are using are natural and completely free of animal products (vegetarian or kosher pareve "nondairy" products, for instance, often contain casein, a milk protein; vegan nondairy products, on the other hand, definitely do not).

Fats—Fat is essential in cooking to impart flavor. When something is too bitter, a little fat evens the taste; too spicy, it cools and calms the heat. The sensation fats add to a meal is one of fullness and richness. Fats are also crucial to the building and protecting of every cell in our body. Whether it comes from nuts and seeds, such as walnut or flaxseed oil, or from fruits, such as olive oil, we recommend using only unrefined and minimally processed (nonhydrogenated) fats and oils. If a recipe calls for stick-style margarine or shortening, be sure to use that and not tub-style spreads.

Flours—Flour is made by finely grinding and sifting grain. Conventionally, flours are made by using huge steel rollers to break down the grain, creating high heat that destroys valuable vitamins and enzymes. The more nutritious option is stone-ground flour, produced by grinding the grain between two slow-moving stones. This process crushes the grain without creating excess heat, leaving the enzymes and vitamins intact. Stone-ground flours can be purchased in health food stores or supermarkets that carry natural foods.

Sea vegetables—Many have discovered the true potential of these nutrient-rich delicacies from the sea commonly referred to as "seaweed." Full of trace minerals, vitamins, protein, and fiber, they are truly worth having in your diet. We use sea vegetables such hijiki, arame, wakame, dulse, agar, and nori. Sea vegetables are already in most everyone's life—in candy and even toothpaste. If you are new to them, try out a few kinds to find the ones that you like. Most of these are available in health or Asian food stores.

Sweeteners—Sugar was once a luxury item only the rich could afford, because it was so scarce and expensive. Sweeteners come in countless forms; we use a variety to create different flavors and textures. All of the sweeteners we use are available at natural food stores. Note that even natural sweeteners, such as agave syrup and honey, still contain various forms of sugar.

Vinegars—For thousands of years, vinegar has been used throughout the world for everything from a beauty aid to a food preservative. Vinegar has a sweet-and-sour flavor. It aids in digestion.

PANTRY ITEMS
LISTED ALPHABETICALLY

Agar (a.k.a. agar-agar)—Made from seaweed. We use agar powder as a gelling agent. It is great for making puddings, frostings, and the traditional health-supportive dessert, kanten. Agar helps to calm inflamed digestion, and to pull together toxins from the intestines and move them out with its mucilage. Agar is tasteless, odorless, and safer to use than its animal counterpart, gelatin. Gelatin is made from ground-up cartilage of pigs and cows, and these parts of the animals have the potential for carrying mad cow disease. Agar is available in flakes, sticks, and powder. The powder dissolves much more easily than the other kinds. 1 tablespoon of agar flakes is equal to 2 teaspoons of agar powder. See the conversion chart on page 21 to use agar in place of gelatin.

Agave [ah-GA-vay]—A natural liquid sweetener extracted from the agave plant. The plant's syrup makes a great substitute for honey or rice syrup. Agave does not significantly raise the blood sugar level in the body, making it a great sweetener for diabetics.

All-purpose flour—All-purpose flour, which is finely ground wheat, comes in two basic forms, bleached and unbleached, which can be used interchangeably. Flour can be bleached either naturally or chemically, but we prefer unbleached organic all-purpose flour.

Apple cider vinegar—Traditionally made from nothing but the juice of freshly pressed apples that has been fermented over a 4- to 6-week period. It has a strong flavor. Apple cider vinegar can help to maintain the proper acid–alkaline balance in the body.

Arame [AR-ah-may]—A sea vegetable that looks similar to hijiki. It has long, thin, dark brown-green strands. Arame has a multitude of nutritional benefits, including helping with many female issues, such as increasing lactation, relieving menstrual pain, and increasing fertility. It also helps to control high blood pressure, and is an excellent source of protein. Tasty and mild, this versatile vegetable is good on salad or as a warm side dish with sautéed carrots, burdock root, and toasted sesame seeds.

Arrowroot—A starchy powder from a tropical tuber that is used for thickening. It is less processed than cornstarch and can be substituted measure for measure for it.

Balsamic vinegar—The best balsamic vinegar is made in Modena, Italy, from the unfermented juice of white grapes and is both sweet and sour.

Barley malt—A sweetener that is half as sweet as honey. It is made from sprouted barley and has a nutty caramel flavor.

Blackstrap molasses—A rich source of minerals and vitamins. As the last possible extraction of cane in the sugar-refining process, it's the richest in nutrients of any sugar product.

Brown rice—A staple for almost half of the world's population. Brown rice is the entire grain with only the outer husk removed. High in fiber and bran, it has a light tan color, a nutty flavor, and a chewy texture.

Brown rice flour—Imparts a lively, nutty flavor to baked goods. It may be used interchangeably with a portion of the wheat flour in any recipe. (Note: In a baking recipe, do not replace *all* the wheat flour with brown rice flour, or the product will not come out as intended.)

Brown rice syrup (Rice malt)—A thick syrup made from cracked brown rice and barley. It has a neutral flavor and is half as sweet as sugar. Used as a sugar substitute in sweets and desserts.

Bulgur wheat—A staple food in the Middle East, this is cracked wheat. Bulgur is high in nutritional value and has a chewy texture. It makes a great salad or side dish.

Canola oil—A processed oil that comes from the rapeseed plant. Currently we use canola oil for baking or for dressings in which we want to add fat but not flavor. This oil is slowly being phased out of our cooking and is being replaced with other flavorless, high heat–tolerant oils such as grapeseed or safflower, oils that produce the same result with less processing.

Capers—The pickled or brined flower buds of a spiny Mediterranean shrub; a pungent, tart condiment.

Carob—A chocolate substitute made from the powdered seed pod of the carob tree. Measure for measure, it contains three times as much calcium as milk and is rich in potassium and vitamins, as well. Unlike chocolate, carob is free of caffeine.

Chickpea flour—This high-protein flour is made from ground hulled and roasted chickpeas. It looks dry, powdery, and almost chalky; the chickpeas add a sweet, rich flavor. Chickpea flour is gluten free.

Chutney—A sweet, spicy, jamlike condiment served with Indian meals. It's made with fruit, often mango; vinegar; a sweetener; and spices, often some form of curry.

Coconut milk—This nondairy milk has a unique smooth texture and rich flavor. It is made from the meat of the coconut; the liquid inside a coconut is coconut water, not coconut milk. We use an unsweetened coconut milk that has no preservatives.

Coconut oil—A wonderful fat. It can be used to produce the same results as butter in baked goods and also is good for high-heat cooking. Many people hesitate to use coconut oil because it is a saturated fat. This is true, but it does not contain cholesterol like other saturated fats. When heated over 240°F, coconut oil does not lose its beneficial properties. The body also assimilates coconut oil more easily than it does other oils, and so this oil is less fattening. Another benefit is that coconut butter contains caprylic acid, a fatty acid that helps in the reduction of candida, a condition of yeast overgrowth in the body. Most coconut butter is semirefined, taking away most of its flavor, but you can purchase unrefined or raw varieties that have a rich coconut taste.

Cornmeal—This grain has been widely used in Native American cooking for thousands of years. Corn flour absorbs more water than other flours and yields a drier, more crumbly product. Cornmeal has a sweet flavor and adds a beautiful golden color to your culinary creations.

Couscous—A tiny pellet of pasta made from semolina flour. Common in North African and Middle Eastern dishes.

Daikon [DI-con]—A large, white Asian radish with a sweet, fresh flavor.

Dates—These fruits provide a completely raw and unprocessed sweetener. There are many types of dates. We mostly use Medjool dates; they are a larger date that provides a sweet caramel taste. Soak dates overnight to soften them. You can use both the dates and their soaking water to sweeten a variety of foods; also, date syrup is available in health food stores.

Dulse—This incredible purple sea vegetable is rich in vitamin A, magnesium, potassium, and B-complex vitamins. Dulse's many health benefits include strengthening the blood, adrenals, and kidneys; it is also helpful in treating herpes. Dulse, with its nutlike taste, is one of the few sea vegetables grown in North America and is not used in Asia. Lightly toasted dulse makes a tasty snack when mixed with nuts. Available in flake form, it's also good sprinkled on a salad. Try adding dulse to rice and vegetables for a nutritional kick.

Egg replacer—Ener-G is the brand name for a powdered combination of starches and leavening agents that bind cooked and baked foods in place of eggs. It's sold in natural food stores. (See also Flaxseeds.)

Evaporated cane juice—Cane juice evaporated down to a free-flowing crystal. It is less processed than granulated sugar and retains more nutrients.

Extra-virgin olive oil—Olive oil is the fat we use most often for cooking. Primarily, we use it to sauté, or for things like hummus, or on raw food plates. Extra-virgin olive oil is the strongest in flavor of any type of olive oil, as it is the first pressing of the olives. If you are cooking at higher temperatures or making foods for which you do not want to impart a specific flavor, there are better alternatives.

Fermented black beans—Whole black soybeans that are fermented, then salted with orange peel and ginger. You can substitute red miso, but fermented black beans are worth the trip to the Asian market.

Flaxseed oil—We use flaxseed oil in recipes that are not cooked. Heat destroys the benefits of this oil. Some of its many benefits include supporting healthy thyroid, adrenal, and hormonal functions. Flaxseed aids in all brain functions and helps maintain healthy nerves, arteries, skin, and hair. Flaxseed oil also helps in breaking down LDL, the "bad" cholesterol, in the body. It is highly perishable; always keep it refrigerated in a dark container, and use within two weeks of purchase. Flaxseed oil can be added to smoothies, raw plates, soy yogurt, or salads.

Flaxseeds (a.k.a. Linseeds)—Tiny, oval-shaped beige seeds. Bland in flavor, they are rich in omega-3 fatty acids and very high in fiber. Sprinkle on prepared dishes and add to baked goods. See conversion chart for how to use flaxseed meal (finely ground flaxseeds) as an egg replacer in baking.

Florida Crystals—The brand name for evaporated cane juice crystals. It is available in organic and nonorganic varieties.

Gluten flour—A high-protein flour made by removing the starch from hard wheat flour. You can use gluten flour to make seitan quickly and easily. It turns a big, messy process into a simple one.

Goji berries—Antioxidant-rich red berries from Tibet. They are available at natural food stores and from online retailers.

Hempseeds—The seeds of the hemp plant. They contain both linoleic and linolenic acid, and a high concentration of complete protein.

Hijiki (a.k.a. Hiziki) [hee-ZHEE-kee]—By far the most popular type of sea vegetable we use. The plump little black strands have a mild flavor. One cup of hijiki contains more calcium than does the same amount of milk. High in iron and B vitamins, hijiki supports a healthy thyroid and is good for stabilizing blood sugar. Hijiki is soaked before using and grows approximately three times in size, so use a large bowl when reconstituting. We serve hijiki cooked in a simple style with garlic, onions, and ginger. It makes a great side dish or can be wrapped in phyllo dough and baked like strudel.

Hummus—A Middle Eastern dip and spread made of chickpeas mashed with lemon juice, garlic, olive oil, and tahini.

Jasmine rice—An aromatic rice from Thailand, comparable to India's Basmati rice.

Kombu—A wide, thick, dark green sea vegetable used in soups and for cooking beans.

Kudzu (Kuzu) [koo-zoo]—A white, starchy powder made from the root of the kudzu plant. Used for thickening soups, sauces, and puddings. Medicinally, it's used to calm headaches and reduce the effects of hangovers.

Maple syrup—The sap from the sugar maple tree that has been boiled until much of the water is evaporated. It is mineral rich and graded according to color and taste; grade A is the lightest, grade C is the darkest. Grade A is commonly used for topping breakfast items, whereas grade B is often preferred for baking, since its depth of flavor lends richness to the finished product.

Millet—A tiny, round, nutritious golden grain that becomes light and fluffy when cooked. It has a bland flavor and easily absorbs the flavors of herbs and spices. Millet is popular in India and China.

Mirin—A sweet Japanese cooking wine made from rice, with a distinctive flavor that's sweet but not cloying. It is colorless but full of flavor.

Miso [MEE-so]—A salty fermented paste made from cooked aged soybeans; used in Japanese cooking. Available in several varieties, some made with grains as well as soybeans; darker varieties tend to be stronger in flavor and saltier than lighter varieties. We use the lighter varieties in our dishes.

Nama shoyu—Raw, unpasteurized soy sauce used in the preparation of raw food recipes. It can be found at health food stores and through online retailers.

Nori [NO-ree]—Paper-thin crispy sheets of pressed sea vegetable. Usually used for Japanese sushi, rolled around rice or crumbled as a garnish. You can wrap almost anything in it for a quick, healthy snack. Most nori is pretoasted, but you can find it raw from specialty stores. Nori contains the highest amount of protein and vitamins C and A of all the sea vegetables. Nori is a good introduction to sea vegetables, and children like it. Try it as a snack for your kitties as well—they go crazy for it.

Nutritional yeast—An inactive yeast that is used as a dietary supplement and a condiment. It has a distinct but pleasant aroma and is yellow in color, and its taste varies from nutty to cheesy. Nutritional yeast is high in protein and B vitamins. It provides vegans with a nonanimal source of vitamin B_{12}.

Oats—A versatile grain that can be used in a variety of recipes. Commonly used as a breakfast cereal, oats also work well in baked goods, or as a binder in burgers and loaves. We use rolled oats in our recipes.

Phyllo (a.k.a. Filo) [FEE-low]—Tissue-thin layers of pastry used in Greek and Middle Eastern dishes, such as baklava.

Quinoa [KEEN-wah]—A round, sand-colored grain with a mild, nutty taste and light texture. Easy to digest, quinoa has the highest protein of any grain; is rich in minerals, vitamins, iron, and amino acids; and has more calcium than milk. The mother grain of the Incas is naturally covered with a bitter substance called saponin that should be removed by washing well before cooking.

Rice malt (see Brown rice syrup)

Rice milk—A dairy-free milk substitute made from rice. You can use it as a replacement for milk in all your recipes. Rice milk comes in a variety of flavors including chocolate and vanilla.

Rice vinegar—A grain-derived vinegar that is low in acid and has a rich, warm flavor.

Sea salt—Comes from evaporated seawater. Coarse or fine-grained, sea salt has a higher mineral content than any other salt, which is why it imparts a saltier taste than other salts do. We used it to make all the recipes in this book.

Seitan [SAY-tan]—A chewy, meatlike, high-protein food made from boiled or baked wheat gluten. Available as a dry mix or prepared frozen or chilled in the deli section. The dough is then cooked in a variety of broths and spices. Seitan will keep in the refrigerator for a week or in the freezer for 3 months.

Sesame butter (see Tahini)

Shiitake [she-TAH-kee] mushroom—A rich, woodsy mushroom with an umbrella-shaped brown cap, used in traditional Japanese cuisine.

Soy milk—A dairy-free milk made from soybeans. Available unsweetened, plain, or with various flavorings, and fortified with added vitamin B_{12} and calcium.

Spelt flour—An ancient red wheat from the Mediterranean, often used for bread. Spelt has an excellent flavor and is a great alternative for people who are allergic to common wheat.

Spike—An all-purpose seasoning blend of thirty-nine herbs, vegetables, and exotic spices. We love the flavor Spike adds to many recipes.

Spirulina—A blue-green algae used as a dietary supplement. It provides a protein with all essential amino acids and is available in powder and tablet forms.

Sucanat—The brand name for an unrefined, unbleached natural alternative to refined white sugar, made by evaporating and granulating sugar cane juice. It retains more vitamins, minerals, and trace elements than does sugar. It can be used in place of brown sugar and is roughly equivalent to the brand-name sugar product Rapadura.

Sun-dried tomatoes—Tomatoes that have been sun dried or dehydrated, producing a chewy texture. Sold either dry or packed in oil, they are rich in flavor and work excellently in raw food. We use the dried form in our recipes.

Tahini [tah-HEE-nee] (a.k.a. Sesame butter)—A thick, smooth paste made from ground sesame seeds, a good source of calcium. A staple of Middle Eastern cuisine.

Tamari [tuh-MAH-ree]—A dark, rich, fermented naturally brewed soy sauce. Tamari is made without the wheat used in most commercial shoyu (soy sauce) brands.

Tamarind paste—A sour, pungent-flavored paste made from the tamarind fruit.

Tempeh [TEM-pay]—A fermented high-protein cultured soybean cake traditionally used in Indonesia, it has a nutty flavor. Tempeh is less processed than tofu, with high enzymatic activity making for easy digestion. All tempeh should be marinated to remove its bitter taste.

Tofu [TOE-foo]—A white curd made from soybean milk. High in protein, tofu comes in silken (soft), firm, and extra-firm varieties, as well as reduced-fat. Silken tofu, wetter and creamier, is best for desserts, sauces, or dips. We use extra-firm tofu for most other purposes. Our favorite brand is Fresh Tofu—it rocks. If you see it, buy it. If you don't, and you live on the East Coast, ask your local natural foods store to carry it.

Udon [OO-don]—Thick Japanese wheat noodles available in Asian food markets and natural food stores.

Umeboshi [oo-meh-BOH-she] paste—A condiment made from Japanese sour plums that are salted, sun dried, aged, and pureed. Contains iron, calcium, minerals, vitamin C, and enzymes; believed to aid digestion. It imparts a salty, sour flavor.

Unbleached all-purpose flour—Made from wheat that is refined of its bran and germ. Unbleached all-purpose flour yields a lighter product than does whole wheat flour and is great for making cakes and cookies.

Vegetable broth powder—Can be used in place of vegetable stock to add a richer, fuller flavor and it's ready in an instant. You can use bouillon cubes in place of the broth powder if it can't be found.

Vital wheat gluten (see Gluten flour)

Wakame [wah-KAH-meh]—A variety of kombu, a flavor-enhancing sea vegetable. Most people are familiar with wakame in miso soup. Some of its amazing nutritional components include calcium and vitamins A and C. It has the incredible ability to bind and remove heavy metals and to reduce sodium. When cooked with beans, it helps to break down the enzymes in the beans and make them more easily digestible. Toasted and ground, wakame can be used in place of salt.

Wasabi [wah-SAU-bee]—A green Japanese radish with a pungent flavor and a sinus-clearing effect. Wasabi powder mixed with water is used to make the fiery green paste that accompanies sushi. Available in specialty markets as a paste, powder, or the fresh root. Beware of mainstream "wasabi" products that contain ordinary horseradish and green dye. Eden brand wasabi powder is additive free.

Whole wheat flour—Made from hard wheat berries, with their germ intact. This flour contains all forty nutrients of wheat; has a rich, full flavor; and creates a denser product than white flour. A softer but still whole-grain milling that we sometimes use is called whole wheat pastry flour (comparable to using cake flour versus all-purpose flour). Please do not substitute regular whole wheat flour for whole wheat pastry flour, or vice versa, as the texture and density of the product may be adversely affected.

Conversion Ideas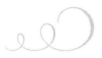

To convert a recipe for a whole-foods vegan diet, try the following substitutions:

Beef	Tofu, tempeh, seitan, or beans
Beef broth	Miso paste or tamari
Butter in baking	Coconut oil
Butter in cooking	Earth Balance brand vegan margarine
Buttermilk	½ cup soymilk mixed with 1 teaspoon lemon juice to curdle the milk
Chicken	Tofu, tempeh, or seitan
Chicken stock	Homemade vegetable stock (page 51) or premade aseptic packaged vegetable broths, powder, or bouillon. Rapunzel makes a great bouillon.
Cornstarch or flour for thickening	Arrowroot powder or kudzu root starch. Substitute in equal measure for the cornstarch. Mix to a slurry in an equal amount of cold liquid before using.
Cream	Coconut milk or soy creamer.
Eggs for binding	Flaxseeds. For one egg, mix 1 tablespoon ground flax meal with 3 tablespoons water to make a slurry.
Eggs for moisture	Applesauce or silken tofu. For one egg, use ¼ cup of tofu or applesauce and a pinch of baking powder.
Eggs for leavening	Ener-G Egg Replacer (see package for amount).
Gelatin	Agar. 1 tablespoon flakes or 1 teaspoon powder to 1 cup liquid.
Mayonnaise	Vegenaise or Nayonaise. These dairy-free alternatives have all the same qualities as mayonnaise, but none of the cholesterol.
Textured vegetable protein	Crumbled lentils or tempeh. You'll get the same effect without all the processing.

Spice Blends

HERB AND
SPICE BLENDS

Most of these blends can be purchased at your local store or online, but if you have the time, freshly preparing your own spice blends is a great way to bring full flavor to any dish. These blends represent some of the most used in our kitchens.

Feel free to experiment with more or less of the herbs and spices you like, rather than keep to the exact measurements in our recipes.

Remember that if substituting dried herbs or spices for fresh, use one-third less of the dried kind; for instance, 1 tablespoon of chopped fresh sage, or 1 teaspoon of dried.

Italian

2 teaspoons each of dried basil, dried marjoram, and dried oregano, plus 1 teaspoon of dried sage.

Mexican or Taco

½ teaspoon of cayenne plus 1 teaspoon each of chile powder, cumin, garlic powder, onion powder, and paprika.

Indian

When putting together Indian spice blends, it enhances the flavor if you gently roast the whole spices in a pan until they release some aroma. Let the spices cool and grind them in a spice grinder. The smells and flavors from this are a wonderful sensory experience.

Curry powder—1 teaspoon each of ground ginger, mustard seeds, and black peppercorns; 2 teaspoons each of coriander seeds, cumin seeds, and ground turmeric; and 1 tablespoon each of curry leaves and fenugreek seeds.

Garam masala—1 teaspoon each of whole cloves and grated nutmeg; 2 tablespoons each of brown cardamom seeds, coriander seeds, cumin seeds, and black peppercorns; and 1 small cinnamon stick, broken up.

Cajun

⅛ teaspoon of ground cayenne; 1 tablespoon each of paprika, white pepper, and thyme; 3 tablespoons each of granulated garlic and black pepper; and ¼ cup of salt.

French

Herbes de Provence—1 teaspoon each of basil, sage, and rosemary; 2 tablespoons of culinary-grade lavender flowers (do not use potpourri lavender); and 3 tablespoons each of oregano and thyme.

Breakfast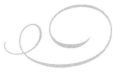

Whether you choose to make Tofu Scramble or Tiffany's Pancakes, breakfast can be a delicious, healthy ritual to start your day. Our Tempeh Sausage and Gravy Biscuits really warm up a winter morning; our Cinnamon Buns are a sweet, decadent treat any time of the year. Try the Papaya Delight for an easy, refreshing meal, or our egg-free version of the brunch favorite, quiche.

The recipes here aren't just for mornings; the Apple Crumb Muffins are a great on-the-go snack, and our granola makes an excellent addition to trail mix for kids.

Apple Crumb Muffins

Yield: 24 muffins

The apples make these muffins moist and light, and the sweet
cinnamon crumb topping is a sensory delight, but they contain
a fraction of the fat of muffins made with milk and eggs.
A delicious combination that is hard to pass up.

Preheat the oven to 375°F. Lightly oil the bases of two 12-compartment muffin tins and insert two dozen cupcake liners. Set aside.

1. In a saucepan, cook the ingredients for the apple mixture over medium heat for 4 to 5 minutes, until just slightly softened.

2. Stir together the ingredients for the crumb topping in a medium-size bowl, being careful not to overmix, and set aside. In a separate, large mixing bowl, stir together all the dry ingredients. In a third, large bowl, stir together all the wet ingredients.

3. Add the wet ingredients to the dry and gently mix until just combined. Gently fold the apple mixture into the batter.

4. Fill the muffin cups three-quarters full and sprinkle each liberally with roughly 1 tablespoon of the crumb topping.

5. Bake for 18 to 22 minutes, turning the pans halfway through the baking process. The muffins are done when a toothpick poked into the middle comes out clean.

VARIATIONS: THESE ARE ALSO DELICIOUS
WITH WALNUTS, ¾ CUP EITHER STIRRED
INTO THE BATTER FOR EXTRA NUTTINESS OR
MIXED INTO THE CRUMB TOPPING FOR
EXTRA CRUNCH.

Apple Mixture
1 tablespoon maple syrup
2 crisp apples (Braeburn or Fuji), peeled, cored, and chopped into small cubes
1 tablespoon canola oil
½ teaspoon ground cinnamon
¼ teaspoon grated nutmeg

Crumb Topping
1¼ cups unbleached all-purpose flour
1 cup uncooked rolled oats
½ cup Sucanat
¼ cup coconut butter or vegan margarine
½ teaspoon vanilla extract
1 teaspoon ground cinnamon
¼ teaspoon grated nutmeg
Pinch of sea salt

Dry Ingredients
2 teaspoons baking powder
2 teaspoons baking soda
2 cups unbleached all-purpose flour
1½ cups whole wheat flour
2 teaspoons ground cinnamon
1 teaspoon ground ginger

Wet Ingredients
1¼ cups canola oil
1½ cups maple syrup
2 tablespoons vanilla extract
1 teaspoon sea salt
2 tablespoons apple cider vinegar
1½ cups water

Banana Bread

Yield: One 9-inch loaf

This simple banana bread is a great way to use up any extra bananas that may be too ripe to eat. Hempseeds provide added protein and an omega-3 punch.

2 cups unbleached
  all-purpose flour
1½ teaspoons baking
  powder
½ teaspoon baking soda
½ cup canola oil
¾ cup Sucanat
½ teaspoon sea salt
¼ cup soy milk
¼ cup maple syrup
1 teaspoon vanilla extract
4 large ripe bananas,
  mashed
½ cup hempseeds or nuts
  of choice, chopped
  roughly

Preheat the oven to 350°F. Lightly oil a 9 by 3-inch loaf pan and set aside.

1. In a large bowl, sift together the flour, baking powder, and baking soda. Set aside.

2. In another bowl, mix together the oil, Sucanat, and salt. Stir in the soy milk, maple syrup, and vanilla. Add the bananas to the mixture and mix well.

3. Add the banana mixture and hempseeds to the dry ingredients, and mix thoroughly.

4. Pour the batter into the prepared pan and bake for 45 to 50 minutes, or until a toothpick poked into the middle comes out clean.

Basic Biscuits

Yield: 12 biscuits

These biscuits are our take on a Southern tradition, and a welcome, easy-to-make addition to a hearty breakfast.

2 cup unbleached
  all-purpose flour
2 teaspoons baking powder
½ teaspoon baking soda
½ teaspoon sea salt
6 tablespoons coconut oil
  or vegan margarine
⅔ cup soy milk
1½ teaspoons lemon juice

Preheat the oven to 350°F. Line a baking sheet with baking parchment.

1. Sift the dry ingredients together into a mixing bowl.

2. Cut the margarine into the flour mixture until it resembles coarse meal. Make a well in the center of the mixture and pour in the soy milk and lemon juice. Mix together until just moistened.

3. Roll out the dough to ½-inch thickness. Cut into 2-inch circles and place the circles on the prepared baking sheet. Reroll the scraps and cut the rest of the dough into 2-inch biscuits.

4. Bake for 8 to 12 minutes, or until golden brown.

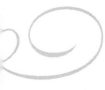

Tempeh Sausage and Gravy Biscuits

Serves 8

Tempeh Sausage
8 ounces Marinated
  Tempeh (page 55)
1½ cloves garlic, minced
1 tablespoon canola oil
2 tablespoons tamari
⅓ teaspoon dried marjoram
Pinch of ground sage
½ teaspoon dried thyme
½ teaspoon paprika
⅛ teaspoon cayenne
¾ teaspoon fennel seeds
Black pepper
¼ cup unbleached
  all-purpose flour
Oil, for coating parchment

Gravy
¼ cup nutritional yeast
½ cup whole wheat flour
2 cups water
2 tablespoons tamari
2 tablespoons extra-virgin
  olive oil
½ teaspoon black pepper

This tasty combo is filled with savory flavors of sage and fennel. The sausage is versatile and easy to prepare and can be made into patties or crumbled. Try it as a delicious topping for pizza. The country gravy is great on mashed potatoes or as a variation to brown gravy, or add it to a soup with seitan and create a hearty country stew.

8 Basic Biscuits (facing page)

Make the Tempeh Sausage:
Preheat the oven to 400°F. Line a baking sheet with baking parchment and brush liberally with oil.

1. Cut the tempeh in half and grate it finely into a large bowl, using a box grater.

2. Add the garlic, canola oil, tamari, the herbs and spices, and the flour. Mix together, then form into 3½-inch patties.

3. Place the patties on the prepared baking sheet and bake for 15 minutes, or until crisped on the outside.

Make the Gravy:
1. Put the nutritional yeast and flour in a 1-quart saucepan and toast over medium heat until light brown.

2. Turn the heat down to very low, and slowly whisk in the oil to form a roux. Gradually whisk in the water and tamari until the gravy is smooth.

3. Raise the heat back to medium and continue cooking, stirring constantly with the whisk until thickened.

TO SERVE: PLACE EACH TEMPEH PATTY ON A BISCUIT AND TOP IT WITH HERB GRAVY.

29

Cinnamon Buns

Yield: 8 buns

Hot, sticky, sweet, soft, cinnamon-infused buns . . . who can resist them? Add raisins or chopped nuts for another variation. Enjoy these scrumptious cinnamon buns with a cup of coffee or tea for a nearly guilt-free breakfast treat.

Preheat the oven to 375°F. Line one large or two small baking sheets with baking parchment and set aside.

1. Mix the yeast and ⅓ cup of the Sucanat in a large mixing bowl.

2. Warm the soy milk over medium heat for 1 to 2 minutes (until it reaches about 104°F on an instant-read thermometer), then add to the Sucanat mixture and let sit in a warm place for 10 minutes.

3. Stir in the coconut oil, add 1 cup of the spelt flour, and mix well. Sprinkle in the salt, then continue gradually adding the spelt flour and mixing until you have an elastic dough that is soft but not sticky. Add the unbleached all-purpose flour in small increments as necessary, to keep the dough from sticking.

4. Knead the dough for 3 to 5 minutes, until it bounces back when pressed lightly with a finger.

5. Transfer the dough to an oiled bowl and let it rest, covered, for 15 minutes or longer, until the dough doubles in size. Punch down and knead the dough for a minute or two, then roll out to a ¼-inch-thick rectangle.

6. Mix together the cinnamon and the remaining ½ cup of Sucanat and sprinkle over the dough with a bit more on the quarter nearest you. Drizzle the maple syrup across the surface of the dough.

Buns
1½ tablespoons active dry yeast

⅓ plus ½ cup Sucanat or brown sugar

1½ cups warm soy milk

¼ cup coconut oil or vegan margarine, melted, at room temperature

1 teaspoon sea salt

2¼ cups spelt flour

¼ cup unbleached all-purpose flour, if needed

½ heaping tablespoon ground cinnamon

¼ cup maple syrup

Glaze
¼ cup powdered Florida Crystals or confectioners' sugar

¼ teaspoon vanilla extract

¼ teaspoon water

¼ teaspoon ground cinnamon

7. Roll the dough evenly from the bottom away from you to create a long tube. Cut the tube into eight rolls. Place the rolls 2 to 3 inches apart on the prepared baking sheet, press down, and let sit for 10 minutes.

8. Bake the rolls until golden, about 10 minutes. Turn pan around and bake for an additional minute.

9. While the rolls are baking, blend the Florida Crystals, if using, in a blender or spice grinder until powdered. Mix with the vanilla, water, and cinnamon to make a glaze.

10. Remove the rolls from the oven and spread the glaze over the buns while still hot.

French Toast

Yield: 8 slices; serves 4

This is a simple way to create a fun breakfast. Use a thick slice of French baguette to soak up the delicious coating, and serve with fresh fruit, a sprinkle of cinnamon, and maple syrup.

2 cups almond milk (page 40)

¼ cup unbleached all-purpose flour

¼ cup canola oil

2 tablespoons nutritional yeast

½ teaspoon sea salt

6 tablespoons maple syrup

1½ teaspoons ground cinnamon

8 slices French baguette or whole-grain bread

Maple syrup or Fruit Sauce (page 182), for serving

1. Whisk together the almond milk, flour, 2 tablespoons of the oil, yeast, salt, maple syrup, and cinnamon in a medium-size mixing bowl.

2. Dip the bread slices into the mixture on both sides until saturated.

3. Heat the remaining 2 tablespoons of oil on a griddle or in a skillet and cook the slices until golden on both sides.

4. Serve hot with maple syrup or fruit sauce.

31

Adam's Ginger-Oat Waffles with Chamomile–Pine Nut Cream and Nectarines

Serves 6

These wheat-free waffles are great topped with whichever in-season fresh fruits suit your fancy. Peaches in the summer and juicy pears in the fall and winter are especially nice.

2 nectarines or other similar fruits, sliced thinly, for garnish

Pinch of ground cinnamon, for garnish

Cream

1½ cups water

½ cup chamomile flowers, fresh or dried

2 whole cloves

1 green cardamom pod

¾ cup pine nuts, lightly toasted

½ cup Sucanat

Pinch of sea salt

Waffles

1½ cups rolled oats

½ cup pine nuts, lightly toasted

2¼ cups water

1 tablespoon extra-virgin olive oil

1 tablespoon ground ginger

½ teaspoon ground cardamom

Pinch of sea salt

⅓ cup Sucanat

Make the Cream:

1. Bring the water for the cream to a boil in a small saucepan. Remove from the heat and add the chamomile, cloves, and cardamom. Let steep, covered, for 10 minutes.

2. Meanwhile, place the remaining cream ingredients in a blender. Strain the chamomile infusion into the blender. Blend at high speed until the cream is smooth.

3. Chill the cream in the freezer while you make the waffles.

Make the Waffles:

1. Preheat a waffle iron. Oil it lightly if it does not have a nonstick finish.

2. While the iron heats, place the oats and pine nuts in a blender and blend at medium speed while gradually adding the water. When the mixture is smooth, blend in the remaining waffle ingredients except for the garnishes.

3. Pour the batter onto the heated waffle iron, and cook according to the manufacturer's directions until golden brown and cooked through.

TO SERVE: DRIZZLE THE WAFFLES WITH GENEROUS SPOONFULS OF THE CREAM, AND TOP WITH THE NECTARINE SLICES AND A PINCH OF CINNAMON.

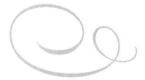

Granola

Yields 8 cups

Dry Ingredients
6 cups rolled oats

1 cup chopped pecans

1 cup pumpkin seeds, chopped into large pieces with a knife

1 cup sunflower seeds

¾ cup hempseeds

2 teaspoons ground cinnamon

¼ teaspoon grated nutmeg

Wet Ingredients
1 cup canola oil

¾ cup maple syrup

½ cup rice syrup

2 teaspoons vanilla extract

¼ teaspoon sea salt

Store-bought cereals are expensive and often not nutritious. Also, commercially prepared granola often contains dairy products. Clusters of oats, nuts, and seeds make this vegan granola rich in calcium, protein, and minerals, and it's very easy to make. Enjoy it with your favorite beverage, sprinkle it over yogurt, or add it to a smoothie. Kids will love it as a snack, too.

Preheat the oven to 350°F. Line two large baking sheets with baking parchment.

1. In a large mixing bowl, stir together the dry ingredients. In a separate mixing bowl, stir together the wet ingredients until well combined.

2. Add the wet ingredients to the dry and mix well.

3. Spread out the mixture on the prepared baking sheets, and bake for 6 minutes. Remove from the oven, stir well, and return to the oven, baking an additional 6 minutes.

4. Remove from the oven and let cool 20 minutes.

5. Will keep stored in an airtight container for several weeks.

Papaya Delight

Serves 2

1 ripe papaya

8 ounces plain or vanilla soy yogurt (we love Whole Soy brand)

½ cup Granola (raw, page 163 or regular, page 33)

This is an easy-to-prepare delight, loaded with simple goodness— enzymes, protein, and live cultures. Topped with our granola, it makes a complete and satisfying breakfast.

1. Slice the papaya in half lengthwise and gently scoop out the seeds with a teaspoon.

2. Fill each hollow with yogurt and top with granola.

CHEF'S TIP: CUT A SMALL SLICE OFF THE UNDERSIDE OF THE PAPAYA HALVES TO HELP THEM LIE FLAT.

Lemon-Blueberry Scones

Yield: 12 scones

These scones are just sweet enough and loaded with blueberries, a great antioxidant-rich food. Make these and you will definitely want to invite friends over for a tea party.

3 cups unbleached all-purpose flour

1 teaspoon salt

1 tablespoon baking powder

½ teaspoon baking soda

½ cup chopped walnuts

2 cups blueberries

¾ cup canola or other flavorless oil

1 lemon, zested and juiced

¼ cup Florida Crystals, plus 2 tablespoons for sprinkling on top

¼ cup maple syrup

¾ cup vanilla soy milk

1½ teaspoons apple cider vinegar

1 tablespoon vanilla extract

1½ teaspoons lemon extract

Preheat the oven to 375°F. Line two baking sheets with baking parchment.

1. In a large bowl, whisk together the flour, salt, baking powder, baking soda, walnuts, and blueberries.

2. In a separate bowl, whisk together the oil, lemon, lemon zest, ¼ cup of the Florida Crystals, and the maple syrup, soy milk, vinegar, and vanilla and lemon extracts, and mix well.

3. Using a rubber spatula, fold the wet mixture into the dry until just combined. Don't overmix.

4. Drop the dough in ¼-cup scoops 2 inches apart onto the baking sheet. Sprinkle with the remaining Florida Crystals.

5. Bake for 20 minutes, or until a toothpick inserted into the center of a scone comes out clean.

Michelle's Blueberry– Sour Cream Coffee Cake

Topping
1 cup whole wheat flour
½ cup Florida Crystals
½ cup vegan margarine, chilled

Cake
¾ cup vegan margarine
1 cup Florida Crystals
¼ cup unsweetened applesauce
1½ teaspoons vanilla extract
2 cups unbleached all-purpose flour
1 teaspoon baking powder
1 cup tofu sour cream
1 cup fresh blueberries

Our friend Michelle loves to bake vegan treats and has generously shared this scrumptious coffee cake recipe, which is as special as she is. Made with tofu sour cream, to give it its moist texture, and juicy blueberries, this cake will be devoured quickly.

Preheat the oven to 350°F. Grease a 9-inch round cake pan and set aside.

Make the Topping:
1. Mix together the whole wheat flour and Florida Crystals.

2. Cut in the vegan margarine until crumbly, and refrigerate the topping until ready to use.

Make the Cake:
1. In a medium-size mixing bowl, cream together the vegan margarine and Florida Crystals. Stir in the applesauce and vanilla.

2. Into a large mixing bowl, sift the flour and baking powder.

3. Add the applesauce mixture and the tofu sour cream to the flour mixture and fold together with a rubber spatula until just mixed. Gently fold in the blueberries.

4. Spread in the prepared cake pan and crumble the topping evenly over the batter.

5. Bake for 30 minutes, or until a toothpick inserted in the center of the cake comes out clean.

Quiche

Yield: One 9-inch quiche; serves 8

This is an appetizing and zesty egg-free version of a Sunday brunch favorite—a light and flaky crust filled with a blend of herbed tofu and spices. Vary the vegetables with the seasons for a change of flavor. This can be cut into smaller bites for a great party food.

Preheat the oven to 400°F.

Coconut Oil Crust

1½ cups unbleached all-purpose flour

½ teaspoon sea salt

1 tablespoon Florida Crystals

¼ teaspoon baking powder

6 tablespoons coconut oil, chilled

¼ cup ice water, or as needed

Quiche Filling

1 (14-ounce) block firm tofu

½ cup nutritional yeast

1 tablespoon tamari

1½ teaspoons white miso

½ teaspoon dried thyme

½ teaspoon dried basil

1 teaspoon sea salt

½ teaspoon black pepper

⅛ teaspoon turmeric

½ teaspoon dry mustard

2 tablespoons extra-virgin olive oil

½ large onion, diced

3 cloves garlic, chopped

½ medium-size zucchini, diced small

½ medium-size carrot, shredded

½ cup broccoli florets, blanched

Make the Crust:

1. Sift together the flour, salt, Florida Crystals, and baking powder. Using a fork or pastry cutter, cut the coconut oil into the flour to form a coarse meal. Add the water slowly until the dough comes together.

2. Roll out the dough and fit into a 9-inch pie plate or tart pan. Lay a sheet of baking parchment over the crust.

3. Weight the bottom of the piecrust with dried beans or uncooked rice, and bake for 10 to 12 minutes, until golden. Remove from the oven, remove the weights, peel off the parchment, and set the crust aside to cool. Turn down the oven temperature to 350°F.

Make the Filling:

1. Crumble the tofu into the bowl of a food processor and process until smooth. Add the nutritional yeast, tamari, miso, thyme, basil, salt, pepper, turmeric, and dry mustard, and blend well. Transfer to a medium-size bowl and set aside.

2. In a sauté pan, heat the oil, add the onion and garlic, and sauté until soft. Add the zucchini, carrot, and broccoli to the pan and sauté, stirring until soft.

3. Add the sautéed vegetables to the tofu mixture and stir until combined.

4. Pour the filling into the prebaked crust and bake for 20 to 25 minutes, until golden brown.

Tempeh Bacon

Yield: 20 slices

3 tablespoons olive oil

2 tablespoons maple syrup

1½ teaspoons tamari

¾ teaspoon liquid smoke

8 ounces tempeh, sliced ⅛-inch thick

A crisp, smoky temptation. The thinner you slice the tempeh and the longer you cook it, the crispier and crunchier it will be. A great breakfast treat, this recipe has many other uses from sandwiches to salads; it stores well and is good to have around.

Preheat the oven to 350°F. Line a baking sheet with baking parchment.

1. Mix all the liquid ingredients together. Brush the bottom of the baking sheet with some of the mixture, then lay the tempeh slices on the sheet. Brush the tempeh slices with the remaining liquid.

2. Bake for 8 to 10 minutes.

Tiffany's Pancakes

Yield: 16 large pancakes

2 cups unbleached all-purpose flour

½ teaspoon sea salt

1½ teaspoons baking powder

½ teaspoon baking soda

½ cup water

¼ cup canola oil

1½ cups vanilla soy milk

1 teaspoon apple cider vinegar

1 teaspoon vanilla extract

¾ cup chopped fruit or nuts

Safflower oil, for the griddle

Vegan margarine, for serving

Maple syrup, for serving

A true classic stands the test of time, and so does Tiffany. A long-time friend and kitchen mate, she shares her love of pancakes with us. These moist and hefty pancakes will make you want to be the first up to surprise the ones you love with these treats.

Preheat the oven to 250°F.

1. Into a large bowl, sift the flour, salt, baking soda, and baking powder.

2. In a medium-size bowl, combine the water, oil, soy milk, vinegar, and vanilla, and whisk until thoroughly combined.

3. Add the wet ingredients to the dry, and whisk until all lumps are gone. Using a rubber spatula, fold in the fruit or nuts.

4. Oil a griddle with the safflower oil and heat over medium heat.

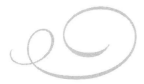

CHEF'S TIPS: KEEP THE
COOKED PANCAKES WARM
ON A FOIL-COVERED PLATE
IN A 250°F OVEN UNTIL
READY TO SERVE.

5. Pour ⅓ cup of batter onto the heated griddle and cook until the underside is golden brown. Flip the pancake with a spatula and cook until the second side is golden.

6. Serve hot with vegan margarine and maple syrup.

For extra-fluffy pancakes, replace the water with ½ cup of seltzer.

Tofu Scramble

Serves 4

The union of tofu and vegetables makes for a tasty breakfast. Create new flavor combinations by adding different seasonal vegetables and spices. The nutritional yeast gives this recipe a rich flavor, and the turmeric adds a bright yellow color.

1 (14-ounce) block firm tofu

3 tablespoons extra-virgin olive oil

1 medium-size onion, diced

3 cloves garlic, minced

1 medium-size red bell pepper, seeded and diced

¾ cup shredded carrot

1 cup diced zucchini

3 tablespoons tamari

¼ cup nutritional yeast

1 teaspoon sea salt

¼ teaspoon Spike

½ teaspoon turmeric

¼ teaspoon paprika

1. Press the tofu according to the instructions on page 95; see its Chef's Tip.

2. In a medium-size sauté pan, heat the oil, then sauté the onions and garlic until soft. Crumble the tofu into the pan, and sauté for 1 minute. Add the remaining ingredients and sauté until the tofu becomes slightly browned.

VARIATION: YOU CAN ALSO PUNCH UP
THE FLAVOR AND NUTRITION BY ADDING
½ CUP OF CHOPPED SPINACH
TOWARD THE END OF COOKING.

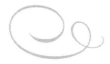

Drinks, Juices, and Smoothies

Juice is a great way to meet your nutritional needs by packing a huge punch of raw, organic fruit and vegetable energy into one glass. It helps to speed up a sluggish metabolism, cleanse the body and blood of toxic cells, and strengthen a weak digestive system. The drinks you'll find here also help to add chlorophyll to your diet, supplying you with essential vitamins and minerals.

This section offers a healthy Immune Booster and also a Heartburn Helper—but don't let those fool you. You'll also find such treats as our scrumptious Root Beer Float, Fruit Slushie, and refreshing Live Lemonade.

Almond Milk

Yield: 4½ cups

1 cup raw almonds
4 cups water
½ teaspoon sea salt
1 vanilla bean, scraped
2 tablespoons raw
   agave nectar

Use this versatile light milk for cereal or in place of rice,
soy, or cow's milk in most recipes. Try substituting
Brazil nuts or cashews for the almonds for a different
flavor and a thicker consistency.

1. Soak the almonds for 6 to 8 hours or overnight. Rinse and drain.

2. In a blender, blend the drained almonds, water, salt, vanilla, and agave on high speed until smooth.

3. Pour the mixture through a fine-mesh strainer into a pitcher, and discard the pulp.

4. Pour the liquid back into the blender and blend well.

This recipe is best used fresh, but will keep for 2 days refrigerated.

Bugs Bunny

Serves 1

1 cup carrot juice
3 scoops vanilla soy ice
   cream
¼ cup crushed ice

Freshly juiced carrot with vanilla soy ice cream and crushed
ice—sweet! This is a beta-carotene-packed Creamsicle in a cup.

1. Pour the carrot juice into a blender and add the ice cream and crushed ice.

2. Blend until smooth.

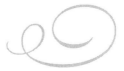

Circulator

Serves 1

A special 2-ounce shot that gets your blood pumping! Liven up a tired body, give a boost to your digestion, or zap that nasty cold.

1 (1-inch) piece fresh ginger
½ lemon
Cayenne
1 ounce flaxseed oil

1. Juice the ginger and lemon into a cup.
2. Add the flaxseed oil and approximately ¼ teaspoon of cayenne (or to taste) to the cup, and stir.

Fruit Slushie

Serves 1

Try this on a hot summer day for a fruit-infused cool-down.

1 cup apple juice
3 frozen strawberries
2 ounces frozen blueberries
1 banana, cut into small pieces

1. Pour the apple juice into a blender.
2. Add the strawberries, blueberries, and banana, and blend until smooth.

CHEF'S TIP: PREPARE FOR SMOOTHIES AHEAD OF TIME BY PLACING THEIR FRUIT INGREDIENTS IN RESEALABLE PLASTIC BAGS AND FREEZING. FROZEN FRUITS MAKE QUICKER, THICKER, SHAKELIKE SMOOTHIES.

Good Ol' Carrot

Serves 1

Carrot juice is a great source of beta-carotene and powerful antioxidants. What a way to start your day!

Approximately 4 medium-size carrots, peeled

Optional Additions
2–3 (1½-inch) pieces beet, peeled
1 (1½-inch) piece fresh ginger, peeled
A handful of greens, washed well
1 small clove garlic
½ apple

1. Juice any optional ingredients first.
2. Run enough carrots through the juicer to bring the juice up to 12 ounces.

Immune Booster

Serves 1

Da Bomb! Tastiest way to get lots of vitamins!

1 small clove garlic

1 (½-inch) piece fresh
ginger, peeled

½ small beet, peeled and
cut into pieces

½ lemon

A handful of greens,
washed well

½ medium-size apple

Approximately 4
medium-size carrots,
peeled

1. Juice the garlic, ginger, and beets, then the lemon.
2. Juice the greens, followed by the apples.
3. Run enough carrots through the juicer to bring the juice up to 16 ounces.

Live Lemonade

Serves 1

The best lemonade we've ever had—fresh organic lemons and apples with a bit of ginger over ice!

½ lemon

1 (½-inch) piece fresh
ginger, peeled

Approximately
4 medium-size apples

4 ounces crushed ice

Optional Additions

3–4 (1½-inch) pieces fresh
beet, peeled

A handful of greens,
washed well

1. Juice the lemon, ginger, and any optional vegetables first.
2. Run enough apples through the juicer to bring the juice up to 12 ounces and add the ice.

Drinks, Juices, and Smoothies

Maegan's Heartburn Helper

Serves 1

2 ounces water
1 teaspoon baking soda

In the olden days before prepackaged medications and 24-hour pharmacies, everybody knew this easy tummy-relief remedy. Now, we proudly pass it down to you. Drink to your health!

1. Stir together in a small shot glass and drink it down. Heartburn's gone!

Root Beer Float

Serves 1

3 scoops vanilla soy
   ice cream
1 (12-ounce can)
   all-natural root beer

Vanilla ice cream floating in luscious root beer is a dream come true in a glass. This is a fun thing to make with the kids on special occasions. It's a great childhood memory of ours.

1. Place the ice cream in a 16-ounce glass.
2. Slowly and carefully pour the root beer over the ice cream.

CHEF'S TIP: BE CAREFUL WHEN POURING SODA OVER SOY ICE CREAM—THE ICE CREAM WILL RISE QUICKLY AND MAY SPILL OVER THE GLASS!

Soy Shake

Serves 1

1 cup soy milk
3 scoops soy ice cream
   (flavor of your choice)

Optional Additions
Strawberries
Blueberries
Peanut butter
Almond butter
Bananas

Just like an old-fashioned shake but without all the dairy. Blend soy milk with your favorite soy ice cream; add fruit, nuts, or peanut butter for an extra-special treat!

1. Pour the soy milk into a blender.
2. Add the ice cream and your desired optional additions, and then blend until smooth.

Strawberry Sunrise

Serves 1

1 cup soy milk, rice milk, or apple juice

4 strawberries

1 banana, cut into small pieces

2 ounces granola (raw, page 163, or regular, page 33)

A healthy breakfast to have on the run. On the many mornings we don't have time to prepare a big breakfast, a shake is a great way to start the day. Use our granola in this recipe—it's packed with all kinds of good stuff.

1. Pour the liquid of choice into a blender.
2. Add the fruit and granola, and blend until smooth.

Spirulina Rush

Serves 1

1 cup apple juice

3 ounces blueberries

1 banana, cut into small pieces

2 ounces hempseeds

1 ounce flaxseed oil

1 tablespoon spirulina

This shake is packed with essential fatty acids and spirulina—a food that is a complete protein. Complete proteins supply you with all the essential and nonessential amino acids that help with all body and brain functions. What a rush!

1. Pour the apple juice into a blender.
2. Add the fruit, hempseeds, and flaxseed oil, and start blending.
3. With the blender running, slowly add the spirulina, and blend until smooth.

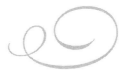

Vegan Nog

Serves 6–8

This wintertime favorite is thick, rich, and creamy—sure to satisfy your most nog-crazed friends! It is a beloved favorite at our holiday parties—we can never make enough.

2 (12.3-ounce) boxes firm silken tofu

1½ cups evaporated cane juice

2 tablespoons vanilla extract

¼ teaspoon ground cinnamon

½ teaspoon sea salt

½ teaspoon freshly grated nutmeg, plus extra for garnish

⅛ teaspoon ground cloves

¼ teaspoon ground ginger

⅛ teaspoon ground cardamom

6 cups vanilla soy milk

⅛ cup grape seed oil

Soy whipped cream, for garnish

1. In a bowl, mix together all the ingredients except the soy milk and oil.

2. Put half of the mixture into a blender and add half of the soy milk. While the mixture is blending, slowly drizzle in 1 tablespoon of the oil to help thicken it. Blend until smooth, and then pour the mixture into a clean bowl. Repeat the process with the other half of the mixture, soy milk, and oil.

3. Whisk together both batches of the ingredients and chill for at least 1 hour.

4. Top with soy whipped cream and some freshly grated nutmeg.

Basics and Sides

From the scrumptious nondairy "cheese" basics to the equally delectable Sesame Yams, you can use these staples and sides your first time in the kitchen or your fiftieth.

Baked Tofu, Marinated Tempeh, and Cashew Rice can be components of a recipe, great jumping-off points for a whole meal, or delicious comfort-food side dishes. Try different combinations or use the House Marinara in an unusual way that you may not have done before. Having any one of these basics on hand can inspire a creative cooking experience.

Cooking Beans

Beans are hearty and delicious and are known throughout the world for their valuable protein. Dried beans need to be washed carefully, as they often include stones. To wash, place the beans in a bowl, fill halfway with water, and swirl around with your hand to loosen any dirt and insects. Pour off all floating debris and floating beans, then catch the rest of the beans in a fine-mesh strainer. If the water still looks dirty, repeat the process.

Most should be soaked before cooking to help minimize gas-producing acids. You don't need to soak lentils, black-eyed peas, split peas, or adzuki beans. Place the beans in a bowl covered halfway to the top with water, and let stand at room temperature for about eight hours. (If you need to soak them for more than eight hours, put them in the refrigerator.) When you're done soaking, drain the beans and rinse well.

Contrary to popular belief, salting beans at the start of cooking does not make them hard and it improves the flavor. It's actually the acid in the cooking water that will slow cooking.

We like to add a 3-inch piece of kombu to the pot at the start of cooking to add flavor and nutrients.

Cooking Grains

Grains are complex carbohydrate foods filled with fiber and nutrition. They are a staple food around the world and an essential part of a vegetarian diet. Rich in minerals and vitamins, they are easy to prepare and can be used in a variety of dishes. The combination of rice and beans creates a complete protein. Grains should be rinsed before cooking.

BEANS (1 CUP DRIED)	CUPS WATER	COOK TIME	CUPS YIELD
Adzuki (Aduki)	4	45–55 minutes	3
Black beans	4	1–1½ hours	2¼
Black-eyed peas	3	1 hour	2
Cannellini (white kidney beans)	3	45 minutes	½
Fava beans, skins removed	3	40–50 minutes	1⅔
Garbanzos (Chickpeas)	4	1–3 hours	2
Great northern beans	3½	1½ hours	2⅔
Green split peas	4	45 minutes	2
Yellow split peas	4	1–1½ hours	2
Kidney beans	2	1 hour	2¼
Lentils, brown	2¼	45 minutes–1 hour	2¼
Lentils, green	2	30–45 minutes	2
Lentils, red	3	20–30 minutes	2–2½
Lima beans, large	4	45 minutes–1 hour	2
Lima beans, small	4	50–60 minutes	3
Mung beans	2½	1 hour	2
Navy beans	3	45 minutes–1 hour	2⅔
Pink beans	3	50–60 minutes	2¾
Pinto beans	3	1–1½ hours	2⅔
Soybeans	4	3–4 hours	3

Chart courtesy of www.vegparadise.com.

GRAIN (1 CUP DRIED)	POT COOKING		PRESSURE COOKING		CUPS YIELD
	CUPS WATER	TIME (MIN)	CUPS WATER	TIME (MIN)	
Amaranth	2	30	–	–	2½
Barley, whole	3	60	2½	60	3½
Barley, pearled	2½	40	2	30	3½
Buckwheat /toasted kasha	3	30	–	–	2½
Cornmeal	4	30	–	–	2½
Corn, hominy	2½	70	2	60	3
Corn, grits	3	20	–	–	3
Job's tears/ pearl barley	3	50	–	–	3
Kamut	3	60	2½	25	3
Millet	3	30	–	–	3½
Quinoa	2	20	1½	60	2¾
Rice, Basmati, brown	1½	40	1	20	3
Rice, Basmati, white	1¼	35	–	–	3
Rice, brown short grain	2	60	1¼	50	3
Rice, brown medium grain	1½	50	1¼	50	3
Rice, brown long grain	1½	50	1¼	40	3
Rice, sweet	1½	30	1¼	25	3
Rice, white	1½	30	1½	20	3
Rye	2½	60	–	–	3
Spelt	3	25	2	50	2½
Teff	3	60	2½	50	3½
Wheat, cracked	3	25	–	–	2¼
Wheat, bulgur red	2	15	–	–	2½
Wheat, bulgur white	1½	10	2	45	2½
Wild rice	1½	50	–	–	4

Basics and Sides

Vegetable Stock

Yield: 1 quart

Making your own vegetable stock is a good way to customize the base flavor of your soups, as well as to use the odds and ends left in your refrigerator. Good-quality organic vegetables make the best stock. When making stock, make sure all your vegetables are thoroughly scrubbed—any dirt will make the stock taste muddy.

2 cups (total) mixed chopped carrots, celery, and onions
1 clove garlic, smashed
½ cup chopped parsley (½ bunch)
1 bay leaf
3 sprigs fresh thyme
8 cups water

CHEF'S TIP: SINCE YOU CAN USE SCRAPS FROM COOKING, DON'T BE AFRAID TO EXPERIMENT WITH NEW VEGETABLE COMBINATIONS. THE ADDITION OF MUSHROOMS MAKES A RICH AND DARK BROTH, AND PARSNIPS ADD ANOTHER SWEET DIMENSION.

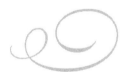

Carrots, onions, and celery are the most commonly used stock ingredients—they create a sweet and neutral-tasting stock. Some vegetables, such as eggplant, collards, bok choy, and other hearty greens, are unsuitable for stocks as cooking them for long periods of time results in a bitter flavor.

Use this stock to make soups or to cook with as a low-fat alternative to oil when sautéing.

1. In a medium or large stockpot, combine the carrots, celery, onions, garlic, and herbs, and cover with water.

2. Bring to a boil, then turn down the heat to a simmer and cook for 25 to 30 minutes over medium heat. If desired, the stock can be simmered longer for a stronger flavor.

3. Strain through a fine-mesh strainer and use immediately, or let cool completely and store for up to a week in the refrigerator or up to 2 months in the freezer.

Baked Tofu

Yield: About 1 pound

¼ cup Basic Marinade (recipe follows)

¼ cup Basic Marinade
(recipe follows)

1 (14-ounce block) firm
tofu, sliced lengthwise
into 8 equal slices

CHEF'S TIP:
MOST TOFU IS SOLD IN
A PLASTIC TUB IN
THE REFRIGERATED
SECTION. THIS IS ABOUT
A POUND OF TOFU,
USUALLY WEIGHING
14 OUNCES.

Baked tofu is a wonderful and versatile recipe. We bake a bunch up ahead of time and keep it in the refrigerator for a quick club sandwich or to top a salad for a little extra protein. Top it with a favorite sauce such as teriyaki or peanut and serve with vegetables and a grain for an easy, satisfying meal.

Preheat the oven to 350°F.

1. Line a baking sheet with baking parchment and brush with a thin layer of the marinade.

2. Place the tofu slices on the baking sheet in a single layer and brush the tops with marinade.

3. Bake for 18 to 20 minutes until golden, rotating the pan halfway through.

Basic Marinade

Yield: Approximately 3¼ cups

1 cup canola oil

1 cup extra-virgin olive oil

3 tablespoons stone-ground
mustard

4 cloves garlic

¾ cup tamari

¼ cup balsamic vinegar

¼ cup fresh lemon juice

1 teaspoon freshly ground
black pepper

Dash of hot sauce

1. Pour all ingredients into a blender and blend until completely mixed.

Will keep for 3 weeks refrigerated.

Basics and Sides

Homemade Seitan

Serves 4–6 (about 4 cups)

Making seitan can be a very messy adventure in the kitchen, but this easy-to-prepare recipe will make you wonder why anyone would do it any other way. Using gluten flour cuts down on the time and mess because the bran has already been washed away.

Seitan Dough

1 cup vegetable broth or water

½ cup unbleached all-purpose flour

1½ cups vital wheat gluten

Cooking Stock

12 cups water

2 tablespoons vegan vegetable-flavor broth powder, or 1 vegan vegetable-flavor bouillon cube

2 tablespoons tamari

1 (1-inch piece) fresh ginger, peeled and chopped roughly

8 cloves garlic

1 medium-size onion, quartered

1 tablespoon Italian seasoning mix (page 23)

Make the Seitan Dough:

1. Pour the broth into a large mixing bowl, then add the all-purpose and gluten flour. Mix just until combined but don't overmix. The dough will be elastic.

2. Divide the dough into two equal-size balls and set aside to rest for 5 to 10 minutes.

3. Slice the gluten rolls into ½-inch slices.

Make the Cooking Stock:

1. Combine all the stock ingredients in a large pot and bring to a simmer. Add the gluten slices and bring back to a boil.

2. Turn down the heat and simmer, uncovered, for 40 to 50 minutes.

3. Remove the gluten slices from the liquid and allow to cool.

You can reserve the stock and store the seitan, in stock to cover, in the refrigerator for up to 1 week or, drained, in the freezer for 2 months.

Marinated Tempeh

Yield: 1 pound

This basic method will remove any bitter taste from the tempeh. Let the tempeh marinate for as long as you wish— the longer, the better.

4 cups water

1 tablespoon extra-virgin olive oil

½ cup tamari

4 cloves garlic, pressed

1 teaspoon spicy mustard

2 tablespoons vegan vegetable-flavor broth powder, or 1 vegan vegetable-flavor bouillon cube

1 (3-inch) piece fresh ginger, cut into disks

1 pound tempeh, cut into 4–6 pieces

1. Put all ingredients in a 4- to 6-quart saucepan and simmer, uncovered, for 15 to 30 minutes, depending on how strongly flavored you wish the tempeh to be.

2. Remove the tempeh from the broth and let cool before using. Reserve the broth for later use.

CHEF'S TIP: MARINATE A FEW PACKAGES OF TEMPEH AT A TIME, FREEZE, AND USE AS NEEDED. IF YOU WANT TO SAVE THE BROTH AND USE IT AGAIN TO MARINATE MORE TEMPEH, YOU CAN FREEZE THAT AS WELL. THE BROTH CAN ALSO BE STRAINED AND USED AS A BASE FOR SAUCES THAT CAN BE SERVED WITH THE TEMPEH, SUCH AS THE CURRY SAUCE FOR THE THAI COCONUT STICKS (PAGE 141).

Carmelized Onions/ Carmelized Leeks

Yield: 1 cup

2 teaspoons extra-virgin olive oil

4 medium-size onions, sliced thinly, or 3 large leeks, white and tender green parts only, well washed and sliced thinly

½ teaspoon sea salt

1. Heat the oil in a sauté pan over medium-high heat. Add the onions and salt and cook, stirring often, until they begin to caramelize and turn golden brown, 10 to 15 minutes.

CHEF'S TIP: TO CLEAN LEEKS, CUT OFF THE TOPS WHERE THE PALE GREEN TURNS DARK AND BEGINS TO FAN AWAY. CUT A LEEK LENGTHWISE FROM THE TOP, STOPPING A HALF INCH FROM THE ROOT. ROTATE THE LEEK A QUARTER TURN AND MAKE ANOTHER CUT, LEAVING THE LEEK ATTACHED AT THE ROOT END. PLUNGE THE LEEK ENDS INTO A BOWL OF COLD WATER, SWISH AROUND, AND RUB THE ENDS TO LOOSEN DIRT AND GRIT. REPEAT UNTIL THE LEEK IS CLEAN.

Basics and Sides

Cashew Rice

Yield: 3½ cups

2½ cups jasmine rice

3 cups water

½ cup dry-roasted cashews

½ cup toasted coconut

½ teaspoon ground cumin

1½ teaspoons extra-virgin olive oil

½ teaspoon sea salt

½ teaspoon ground cinnamon

1. In a medium-size pot, bring the water and rice to a boil. Cover, turn down the heat to a simmer, and cook for 15 minutes.

2. Add the remaining ingredients and mix well.

Bread Sticks

Yield: 12 breadsticks; serves 6

1 teaspoon active dry yeast

1½ cups warm water, roughly 104°F

1 teaspoon Sucanat

1 teaspoon dried dill

½ teaspoon dried thyme

¼ teaspoon dried basil

2 tablespoons extra-virgin olive oil, plus extra for oiling bowl

2¼ teaspoons sea salt

3¾ cups unbleached all-purpose flour

1. Combine the yeast, water, and Sucanat in a bowl and set aside in a warm place for about 10 minutes to let rise. Add the herbs.

2. Add 2 tablespoons of the olive oil and the salt, then slowly add the flour until the dough comes together and is soft but no longer sticky. Transfer the dough to a clean, lightly floured surface.

3. Knead the dough for 5 to 10 minutes, until smooth. Place the dough in a lightly oiled bowl, turning the dough over so that the oil coats all sides of the dough. Cover with plastic wrap and let sit in a warm spot until the dough has doubled in volume.

4. Preheat the oven to 375°F. Line a baking sheet with baking parchment.

5. Punch down the dough and knead for 2 to 3 minutes. Divide the dough into twelve balls. Roll out the balls into ½-inch-thick sticks and place on the prepared baking sheet.

6. Bake for 8 to 10 minutes, until golden.

These bread sticks can be frozen and reheated. The baked bread sticks will keep for 2 to 3 days in an airtight container.

Corn Bread

Serves 8

The variations on this recipe are endless: you can punch up the flavor by adding any of the optional ingredients.

1 cup whole-grain cornmeal

½ cup whole wheat pastry flour

½ cup unbleached all-purpose flour

2 teaspoons baking powder

1 cup soy milk

⅓ cup canola oil

⅓ cup maple syrup

½ teaspoon sea salt

Optional Additions

1 cup soy cheese

¼ cup minced jalapeño

¼ cup finely chopped tomato

½ scallion, chopped finely

Preheat the oven to 350°F. Grease a 9-inch round cake pan, a pie dish, or a cast-iron skillet.

1. In a mixing bowl, combine the cornmeal, flours, and baking powder.

2. In a separate bowl, combine the soy milk, oil, maple syrup, and sea salt.

3. Add the wet ingredients to the dry and stir until the batter is smooth.

4. Pour into the prepared pan and bake for 12 to 15 minutes, until the corn bread is golden brown.

VARIATION: FOR BLUEBERRY AND CORN MUFFINS, MIX IN ½ CUP OF BLUEBERRIES AND BAKE IN MUFFIN CUPS FOR 12 MINUTES OR WHEN PRICKED WITH A KNIFE, THE KNIFE COMES OUT CLEAN. SOMETIMES BAKING CAN TAKE A LITTLE LONGER WHEN THE OVEN TEMPERATURE IS NOT THE SAME THROUGHOUT THE WHOLE OVEN.

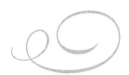

House Marinara

Yield: 3 cups

⅓ cup extra-virgin olive oil

6 cloves garlic, minced

1 medium-size onion, chopped

24 ounces canned whole tomatoes and their liquid

1 cup chopped fresh basil, or 2 tablespoons dried

1 teaspoon dried oregano

1 teaspoon dried rosemary

1 tablespoon maple syrup

1 teaspoon sea salt

½ teaspoon black pepper

1. In a large pot, heat the oil over medium-high heat, add the onion and garlic, and sauté until soft.

2. Add the tomatoes, basil, oregano, rosemary, and maple syrup, and cook over medium heat for 40 minutes, stirring often.

3. Remove from the heat and season with salt and pepper.

4. Allow to cool for a few minutes, then blend the mixture in a blender or food processor until smooth.

Mushroom Gravy

Yield: 3½ cups

1 tablespoon extra-virgin olive oil

½ medium-size onion, diced

2 cloves garlic, minced

1 tablespoon dried thyme

1 tablespoon dried rosemary

1 pound button mushrooms, sliced

1 tablespoon vegan broth powder, or 1 vegan bouillon cube

¾ cup plus 2 tablespoons water

¼ cup tamari

2 tablespoons kudzu

⅓ cup water

1. In a large pot, sauté the onion, garlic, thyme, and rosemary in the olive oil until the onions are soft. Add the mushrooms and cook until they have released their juices.

2. Mix the broth powder and the water together and add to the pot along with the tamari. Bring to a simmer, and cook for 15 minutes.

3. Make a slurry from the kudzu and the remaining water, and add that to the pot. Cook the gravy until it has thickened.

Will keep for 4 to 5 days refrigerated.

Peanut Sauce

Yield: 2 cups

1 cup peanut butter

3 cloves garlic

¼ cup water

¼ cup plus 1 tablespoon
   tamari

Pinch of cayenne

1 (2.1-ounce) package
   Eden Pickled Ginger
   with Shiso, with liquid,
   leaf removed

1. Place all ingredients in a blender or food processor and blend well.

Will keep for 4 to 5 days refrigerated.

**VARIATION: INSTEAD OF USING PICKLED GINGER, YOU CAN ADD
1 TABLESPOON OF FINELY GRATED FRESH GINGER, 2 TABLESPOONS
OF AGAVE SYRUP, AND 1 TABLESPOON OF RICE VINEGAR.**

Nutro Cheese

Yield: 1 pint

2 tablespoons canola or
   other flavorless oil

¼ cup unbleached
   all-purpose flour

Pinch of turmeric

Pinch of cayenne

¾ teaspoon dry mustard

¼ cup soy milk

1¼ cups water

½ tablespoon tamari

¼ cup nutritional yeast

Salt and pepper

*Serve with Philly Seitan Sandwich, over nachos, with tater skins,
or melted atop an Earth Burger for the ultimate Uncheese Burger!*

1. Warm the oil in a small saucepan over medium heat. Whisk in the flour, turmeric, cayenne, and mustard until smooth, then whisk in the soy milk.

2. Add the water and tamari and let cook for 5 to 8 minutes, whisking constantly. Add the nutritional yeast and let cook, whisking, for another 5 minutes or until the mixture is thick. Season to taste with salt and pepper.

Will keep for 4 to 5 days refrigerated.

Sprinkle "Cheese"

Yield: 2 cups

1 cup walnuts, ground finely

1 cup nutritional yeast

½ teaspoon sea salt

1. Process the walnuts and yeast in a food processor until well mixed.

Will keep for 1 month refrigerated, 3 months frozen.

Tofu Cheese

Yield: 4 cups

1 medium-size onion, diced

7 cloves garlic, smashed

2 tablespoons extra-virgin olive oil

2 (14-ounce) blocks extra-firm tofu, crumbled

⅓ cup miso

¼ cup umeboshi paste, or 3 tablespoons brown rice vinegar

1½ teaspoons dried basil

1½ teaspoons dried oregano

1½ teaspoons dried rosemary

1 tablespoon dried parsley

1. In a pan, sauté the onion and garlic in the oil over medium-low heat until they are soft and the garlic can be easily mashed. Transfer to the bowl of a food processor.

2. Add the tofu to the garlic and onion, then mix in the miso, umeboshi, and herbs, and blend until smooth.

Will keep for 2 to 3 days refrigerated.

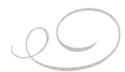

Tofu Sour Cream

Yield: 2 cups

1 (14-ounce) block firm
  tofu
3 tablespoons plus 1
  teaspoon fresh
  lemon juice
3 tablespoons plus
  1 teaspoon canola oil
1 teaspoon brown rice
  vinegar
1 teaspoon sea salt

**Optional Additions
(add only one)**
1 tablespoon fresh dill
1 tablespoon fresh
  rosemary
1 tablespoon fresh basil
1 tablespoon fresh mint
1 tablespoon hot sauce

1. Crumble the tofu into a food processor.

2. Add the lemon juice, canola oil, vinegar, and salt, and whichever optional addition you wish, if using.

3. Process, scraping down the sides of the container with a rubber spatula, until the mixture is smooth.

Will keep for 2 to 3 days refrigerated.

CHEF'S TIP:
USING BOTTLED LEMON JUICE WILL MAKE A MORE
SOUR "SOUR CREAM." YOU WILL NEED ONLY
3 TABLESPOONS IF USING BOTTLED.

Mashed Potatoes

Serves 4–6

4 large russet potatoes,
  peeled and cubed
2 tablespoons extra-virgin
  olive oil
2 tablespoons unsweetened
  soy milk
2 teaspoons sea salt
½ teaspoon black pepper,
  or to taste

1. In a large pot, put the potatoes in enough salted cold water to cover and bring to a boil over high heat.

2. Cook until the potatoes are tender, about 15 minutes. Drain and return the potatoes to the pot.

3. Add the oil, soy milk, and salt and pepper to taste. Mash by hand with a potato masher or fork to the consistency you desire.

4. Serve immediately.

CHEF'S TIP:
NEVER USE A FOOD PROCESSOR OR HAND BLENDER
TO MASH POTATOES! (UNLESS YOU WANT TO MAKE SPACKLE.)

VARIATIONS:
YOU CAN PUNCH THESE
UP A NOTCH BY ADDING
2 TABLESPOONS OF
CHOPPED GARLIC OR
½ CUP OF CHOPPED
SAUTÉED GREENS.

Slow-Cooked Scalloped Potatoes

Serves 6–8

There is no better comfort food than potatoes. This creamy version of an old classic is perfect alone or as part of any feast.

¼ cup extra-virgin olive oil

2 large onions, chopped finely

4 cloves garlic, chopped finely

2 stalks celery, sliced paper thin

4 tablespoons vegan margarine

½ cup unbleached all-purpose flour

2 cups plain soy milk

2 tablespoons tamari

1 tablespoon dried dill

2 teaspoons dried thyme

1 teaspoon sea salt

½ teaspoon black pepper

10 medium-size potatoes, sliced thinly

1 tablespoon paprika

2 tablespoons nutritional yeast

Preheat the oven to 375°F.

1. In a medium-size saucepan, warm the olive oil over medium heat, then sauté the onions, garlic, and celery until the onions and celery are tender.

2. Add the margarine to the vegetable mixture and let melt. Mix in the flour, stirring constantly for 2 to 3 minutes, until you have a dry, lightly browned mixture.

3. In a small bowl, mix together the soy milk, tamari, dill, thyme, salt, and pepper, then add to the saucepan. Stir until well mixed and there are no flour lumps. Set the mixture aside.

4. Lightly oil a 9 by 13-inch baking dish. Pour in ¼ cup of the sauce, then add a layer of potatoes, and alternate layers of potatoes and sauce. Top with paprika and nutritional yeast.

5. Cover and bake for 60 minutes. Remove the cover and bake for an additional 30 minutes, or until potatoes are soft.

Cajun-Spiced Baked Potato Fries

Serves 4

These spiced potatoes are coated with a zesty peppery flavor.
Serve them with the Philly Seitan sandwich or just about
anything. They are sure to satisfy.

2 pounds red potatoes,
   washed, and cut into
   6–8 long wedges
2 teaspoons Cajun
   seasoning mix (see
   Spice Blends, page 24)
1 teaspoon Spike
½ teaspoon garlic powder
A pinch of freshly
   ground pepper
3 tablespoons extra-virgin
   olive oil
Sea salt

Preheat the oven to 425°F. Line a large cookie sheet with baking parchment.

1. In a large mixing bowl, combine the potatoes, Cajun spices, Spike, garlic powder, pepper, and oil, and toss to coat well.

2. Spread out on the prepared cookie sheet.

3. Bake for 40 minutes, turning the pan around in the oven halfway through the cooking time, until the fries are crispy on the edges.

4. Remove the fries and salt to taste.

Mashed Coconut Yams

Serves 4–6

Adding a little coconut milk gives these yams a tropical flavor.
They make a unique, comforting side dish for any meal.

6 cups peeled and diced
   yams
Sea salt
¼ cup coconut milk
2 teaspoons maple syrup
Pinch of nutmeg
Freshly ground black
   pepper

1. In a medium-size pot, put the yams in enough water to cover, and add a pinch of salt.

2. Bring the yams to a boil, then turn down the heat to a simmer and cook for about 20 minutes, or until the yams are tender but not falling apart.

3. Drain the yams in a colander, and let sit for 2 minutes until the water is completely drained.

4. With a fork, mash the yams with the coconut milk, maple syrup, nutmeg, and salt and pepper to taste until the ingredients are well incorporated but the mixture is not too smooth.

Roasted Yams

Serves 6

You can't go wrong with the basic yam,

sure to be delicious every time.

5 large yams, peeled and cubed

2 tablespoons extra-virgin olive oil

2 teaspoons dried thyme

2 teaspoons sea salt

Preheat the oven to 400°F. Oil a baking sheet.

1. Place the cubed yams in a bowl, add the oil, sprinkle with thyme, and toss to coat.

2. Turn out onto the prepared baking sheet, and roast in the oven until softened and browned, about 25 minutes.

3. Remove yams from the oven and sprinkle with salt to taste.

Sesame Yams

Serves 4

A sweet, caramelized, sesame treat—always a hit. Serve it

as a hot side with any Asian or Caribbean entrée.

4 medium-size yams, peeled and sliced into ¼-inch rounds

¼ cup extra-virgin olive oil

¼ cup maple syrup

¼ cup sesame seeds

1 pinch sea salt

Preheat the oven to 400°F. Line two large baking sheets with baking parchment, and lightly oil.

1. In a 6-quart stockpot, bring water to a boil, and add the yams. Cook for 5 minutes, until the yams are slightly tender; drain well.

2. In a mixing bowl, toss the yams with the olive oil and transfer to the prepared baking sheets. Bake for 20 minutes, until the yams start to soften.

3. Remove from the oven and pour the maple syrup over the yams. Return the pans to the oven for 10 minutes, rotating the pans halfway through the baking process. Remove from the oven when the syrup has thickened and caramelized.

4. Meanwhile, toast the sesame seeds in a dry skillet until golden, stirring the seeds to toast them evenly.

5. Sprinkle the seeds over the baked yams and season lightly with sea salt.

6. Remove from the parchment and serve.

Sautéed Greens

Serves 4–6

1 tablespoon extra-virgin olive oil

3 cloves garlic, chopped

1 bunch kale or other greens, washed well, stemmed, and chopped (roughly 4–6 cups)

¼ cup water

1 teaspoon tamari

In the age of quick, microwaved frozen vegetables, this simple, classic dish has fallen by the wayside. Healthful and delicious, dark greens have most of the nutrients your body is clamoring for, and a taste that is savory heaven. Even if you've never had them before, pick up a bunch of greens (kale, chard, collards, mustard greens, beet greens, and so on) from your grocer or local farmers' market and try them—you'll be glad that you did!

1. In a large sauté pan over medium-high heat, heat the oil and then sauté the garlic for 2 minutes.

2. Add the chopped kale, water, and tamari, and cook down until the greens have softened, 5 to 7 minutes.

Note that more delicate greens (spinach, beet greens, chard) will cook quickly, whereas heartier varieties will cook for 20 minutes or more.

Pickled Vegetables

Yield: 3 cups

2 tablespoons pickling spice

Enough water to cover

6 tablespoons apple juice

½ cup rice vinegar

3 cups vegetables (see below)

Pickled Beets
3 large beets, julienned

Pickled Carrots
3 cups matchstick-sliced carrots

Pickled Onions
3 cups sliced onions and ¼ teaspoon turmeric

Pickled Red Cabbage
3 cups chopped red cabbage

Pickling vegetables is a tasty but nearly forgotten kitchen art.

1. Wrap the pickling spices in a piece of cheesecloth secured with kitchen string. Place in a large pot with the water, juice, vinegar, and the vegetable of choice, and bring to a boil.

2. Remove from the heat and let cool. Store the vegetables in their cooking liquid to cover in a tightly lidded jar and place in the refrigerator.

Will keep for 2 to 3 weeks.

65

Soups

Soup is pretty foolproof—perfect for beginning cooks. It's a great food to pull together with whatever you have on hand, especially grains and beans. You can also use the best seasonal offerings to make something special, such as gazpacho or a bright, fresh veggie medley. A creamy soup doesn't have to be dairy-based; pureeing or adding potatoes, other root vegetables, or coconut milk can create the same velvety textures and opaque appearance that cream can—and you won't miss the dairy.

These recipes are simple and to the point, many using carrots and onions as a base. Prepare these recipes in big batches and freeze them for later, or drop some off to share with a friend. All of these soups can be made in advance and reheated.

Black Bean Soup

Serves 4–6

2 tablespoons extra-virgin olive oil

1 large onion, cut in medium-size dice

1 medium-size carrot, chopped roughly

1 small sweet potato, chopped roughly

2 stalks celery, chopped roughly

8 cloves garlic, chopped roughly

2 (15-ounce) cans black beans, drained and rinsed well, or 4 cups precooked

2 tablespoons mild chile powder

1 chipotle, seeded and chopped

1 (14-ounce) can diced tomatoes

Sea salt

Tamari

1 tablespoon tofu sour cream, for garnish

Chopped fresh tomato, for garnish

This soup is hearty black bean goodness. We use canned beans in this recipe so it doesn't take long to prepare, but feel free to soak and cook the beans yourself, if you prefer. (We advise that you cook them before adding them because otherwise the soup would take more water than specified.) For an extra kick, add a few dashes of hot sauce and a squeeze of fresh lime. This soup is beautiful served with some finely chopped red onion, tofu sour cream, and a wedge of golden corn bread.

1. In a 4- to 6-quart stockpot, heat the oil and sauté the onions, celery, sweet potatoes, carrots, and garlic until softened and beginning to brown. Add the black beans and chile powder, and add enough water to cover. Bring to a boil, then turn down the heat to a simmer. Cook, uncovered, for an hour, adding more water if necessary.

2. When the beans are soft, add the chipotle and blend, either in batches in a regular blender or with an immersion blender.

3. Season to taste with the sea salt and tamari.

4. Mix in the canned tomatoes and cook until they are heated through. Top with the tofu sour cream and chopped fresh tomatoes.

Soups

Curried
Red Lentil Soup

Serves 4–6

Spicy, warming, and thick, this Indian-inspired soup is flavored with cinnamon, curry, and mustard seeds. Serve it with a big salad and crusty bread.

2 tablespoons extra-virgin olive oil

2 medium-size red onions, cut into medium dice

½ teaspoon minced garlic

2 stalks celery, cut into medium dice

1 medium-size carrot, cut into medium dice

1 medium-size sweet potato, cut into small dice

2 teaspoons mustard seeds

1 tablespoon curry powder

½ teaspoon ground cinnamon

1 teaspoon ground cumin

1 tablespoon ground ginger

½ teaspoon ground coriander

1 tablespoon minced fresh ginger

1½ teaspoons seeded and minced fresh red chile

½ teaspoon turmeric

1½ cups dried red lentils, washed and picked over

8 cups water

¼ cup maple syrup

½ cup tamari

½ teaspoon salt

½ teaspoon pepper

Minced fresh parsley, for garnish

Minced fresh cilantro, for garnish

1. In a medium-size pot, over medium heat, sauté the onions, garlic, celery, carrots, and sweet potato in the olive oil for 3 minutes. Add the spices and sauté with the vegetables.

2. Add the lentils and stir to mix. Add the water and cook, uncovered, for approximately 30 minutes over medium heat, stirring frequently to prevent sticking, until the lentils are soft.

3. Season the soup with the maple syrup, tamari, salt, and pepper. Sprinkle with fresh minced parsley and cilantro.

CHEF'S TIP:
THIS SOUP CAN BE SERVED
EITHER CHUNKY
OR PUREED UNTIL SMOOTH.

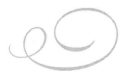

70

Coconut-Squash Soup

Serves 6

*This velvety soup is as decadent as any cream-based soup,
but without the cholesterol, calories, or guilt.*

1 medium-size onion, cut into medium dice

2 stalks celery, chopped

1 medium-size carrot, peeled and chopped

2 tablespoons extra-virgin olive oil

4 cups butternut squash (1 medium-size squash) or yams, peeled and chopped

4½ cups water

1 (15-ounce) can coconut milk

3 tablespoons maple syrup

Salt and pepper

1. In a 4- to 6-quart stockpot, sauté the onions, celery, and carrots in the olive oil for about 5 minutes or until soft. Add the squash and coat with the oil. Add the water and bring to a simmer, making sure to stir the bottom of the pot. Let cook, uncovered, until the squash is soft.

2. Stir in the coconut milk and maple syrup, then blend in batches in a regular blender or with an immersion blender until smooth.

3. Season to taste with salt and pepper.

Gazpacho

Serves 6–8

*It's never too hot for soup. Take advantage of the jewels of
your summer garden, or head out to your local farmers' market
and gather what the sellers have to offer. You can add any of
your favorite vegetables to the mixture.*

6 medium-size fresh tomatoes, cored and diced

1 medium-size red onion, peeled and diced finely

2 cucumbers, peeled, seeded, and diced

1 large red bell pepper, seeded and diced finely

½ cup fresh lemon juice

¼ cup tamari

2 tablespoons hot sauce

½ teaspoon sea salt

1 cup fresh or frozen corn kernels

½ cup finely chopped fresh cilantro

½ cup finely chopped fresh basil, or 1 tablespoon dried

½ cup finely chopped fresh parsley, or 1 tablespoon dried

1. Combine the diced tomatoes, onion, cucumbers, and bell pepper in a large bowl.

2. Add the lemon juice, tamari, hot sauce, and salt.

3. Put half of the mixture into a blender and blend for 30 seconds on medium speed until finely textured.

4. Combine the blended mixture with the diced mixture and add the corn. Stir in the cilantro, basil, and parsley.

5. Cover and refrigerate until chilled.

TO SERVE: FOR A NICE TOUCH, TOP WITH FRESH AVOCADO SLICES, SCALLIONS, OR TOFU SOUR CREAM (PAGE 61).

Soups

Mediterranean Lentil Soup

Serves 8

This soup is simple, fast, and delicious.

2 tablespoons extra-virgin olive oil

4 medium-size carrots, cut into medium dice

3 stalks celery, cut into medium dice

1 large red onion, cut into medium dice

4 cloves garlic, minced

2 tablespoons Italian seasoning (see page 23)

2 cups dried lentils, washed and picked over

12 cups water

½ cup tamari

2 cups tomato sauce

Salt and pepper

1. In a 6-quart stockpot, sauté the onions, carrots, celery, garlic, and Italian seasoning in the oil over medium heat for 5 minutes.

2. Add the rinsed lentils and 8 cups of the water and cook until the lentils soften, approximately 20 minutes. Add the remaining 4 cups of water and cook for an additional 15 minutes.

3. Add the tamari and tomato sauce and cook for 10 minutes. Season to taste with salt and pepper.

Potato-Leek Soup with Lemon and Dill

Serves 4–6

The lemon and dill we add to this traditional soup gives it a lightness and zip that's missing in the country classic.

¼ cup extra-virgin olive oil

6 stalks celery, chopped

1 medium-size white onion, cut into small dice

3 cloves garlic, minced

2 small leeks, sliced thinly

2 medium-size potatoes, peeled and cut into small dice

¼ cup vegan vegetable-flavor broth powder, or 2 vegan vegetable-flavor bouillon cubes, dissolved in 6 cups water

3 sprigs fresh dill, chopped, or 1 teaspoon dried

1 lemon, sliced thinly, for garnish

Salt and pepper

1. In a 4- to 6-quart stockpot, sauté the celery, onion, garlic, and one leek in 2 tablespoons of the olive oil until softened.

2. Add the potatoes and broth, and bring to a boil. Turn down the heat to a simmer and cook until the potatoes are soft, approximately 15 minutes. Season to taste with salt and pepper.

3. In a separate pan, sauté the remaining leek over medium-low heat in the remaining 2 tablespoons of oil until crisp but not burned.

4. Garnish each bowl of soup with some dill, the crisped leeks, and a lemon slice.

CHEF'S TIP: IF YOU WANT A THICKER CONSISTENCY, BLEND HALF THE SOUP IN A BLENDER BEFORE GARNISHING.

Three-Bean Chili

Serves 4–6

Our version of chili is hearty and satisfying without the meat.
Try mixing and matching your favorite beans and different
vegetables, for a change of pace.

1 large onion, diced

12 cloves garlic, minced

2 tablespoons extra-virgin olive oil

4 ounces Marinated Tempeh, crumbled (page 55)

3 tablespoons chile powder

4½ teaspoons ground cumin

1 tablespoon dried oregano

1 tablespoon Spike

16 ounces canned tomatoes, or 4 fresh tomatoes, diced

6 cups tomato sauce

1½ cups cooked black beans, or 1 (15-ounce) can, drained and rinsed

1½ cups cooked black-eyed peas, or 1 (15-ounce) can, drained and rinsed

1½ cups cooked pintos beans, or 1 (15-ounce) can, drained and rinsed

½ cup green bell pepper, or 2 roasted red peppers, seeded and diced

½ cup fresh or thawed frozen corn kernels

½ cup tamari

Salt and pepper

1. In a 4- to 6-quart stockpot, sauté the onion and garlic in the olive oil until softened. Add the crumbled tempeh and sauté until lightly browned. Add all the spices and sauté over medium heat for 3 to 5 minutes.

2. Add the tomatoes and tomato sauce. Stir together and bring to a simmer. Add the beans and vegetables, and stir well. Cook over low heat, stirring occasionally to prevent sticking, for 20 to 25 minutes.

3. Add the tamari, and salt and pepper to taste, and cook an additional 5 minutes.

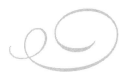

Quinoa-Vegetable Soup

Serves 6

Quinoa is an ancient grain high in protein. Add all of the season's harvest to create this colorful and flavorful soup. Serve it with a salad and it makes a meal.

2 carrots, peeled and diced

4 stalks celery, diced

1½ medium-size onions, diced

4 cloves garlic, minced

3 tablespoons extra-virgin olive oil

2 small yams, peeled and diced

8 cups hot water

2 tablespoons vegan vegetable-flavor broth powder, or 1 vegan vegetable-flavor bouillon cube

½ cup quinoa, well rinsed

1 medium-size summer squash, diced

½ cup spinach, well washed and chopped

1. In a 4- to 6-quart stockpot, sauté the onions, celery, carrots, garlic, and yams in the oil over medium heat for 8 to 10 minutes.

2. Dissolve the broth powder in the hot water, pour over the softened vegetables, and bring to a simmer.

3. Add the quinoa to the pot. Let cook until the quinoa starts to plump and soften, about 15 minutes.

4. Add the squash and spinach at the end of the quinoa cooking time, and cook just until the vegetables are softened and wilted.

5. Season to taste with salt and pepper.

Split Pea Soup

Serves 6

This hearty soup is simple to make and will be a favorite of your whole family at any time of year.

2 small yellow onions, diced

2 small carrots, peeled and diced

2 stalks celery, diced

4 cloves garlic, minced

3 tablespoons extra-virgin olive oil

1½ cups split green peas, rinsed and sorted

2 small russet potatoes, peeled and chopped

10 cups water

½ cup tamari

1 teaspoon liquid smoke flavoring

¼ teaspoon sea salt

¼ teaspoon pepper

1. In a medium-size pot, sauté the onions, garlic, carrots, and celery in the oil for about 5 minutes, or until slightly softened.

2. Stir in the split peas and potatoes. Add 6 cups of the water and simmer for about 20 minutes, stirring frequently to prevent sticking.

3. Add 2 more cups of the water and continue to cook for 15 minutes, or until the peas start to soften. Add the last 2 cups of water and let the soup cook for about 10 more minutes, stirring constantly, until the peas are completely softened.

4. Season the soup with the tamari, liquid smoke, salt, and pepper.

Sweet Potato–Tomato–Chipotle Soup

Serves 6

A great soup for frigid weather, it takes the chill off

on a cold winter's day.

2 tablespoons extra-virgin olive oil

1 large red onion, diced

3 cloves garlic, chopped

2 stalks celery, sliced

3 carrots, peeled and sliced

3 large sweet potatoes, peeled, quartered, and sliced thickly

1 (14-ounce) can diced tomatoes, or fresh

4 cups vegan vegetable stock (page 52) or water

½ cup maple syrup

2 chipotle

2 teaspoons sea salt

1. In a heavy 6-quart stockpot over medium heat, heat the olive oil. Add the onion and garlic, and cook for 3 to 5 minutes. Add the celery and carrots, and cook until softened.

2. Add the sweet potatoes, tomatoes, and stock, and bring to a boil. Turn down the heat and simmer for 30 to 40 minutes, or until all the vegetables are softened.

3. Add the maple syrup, chipotle, and salt.

4. Puree until completely smooth, either with an immersion blender or in batches in a regular blender.

CHEF'S TIP: NEVER FILL A BLENDER MORE
THAN HALFWAY WHEN PUREEING HOT FOODS.
YOU'LL AVOID SOME PAINFUL BURNS!

Soups

Thai Veggie Soup

Serves 6–8

Your friends and family will go crazy for this flavorful soup
packed with lots of colorful vegetables.

2 tablespoons untoasted
    sesame oil

1 small yellow onion,
    minced

4 cloves garlic, sliced thinly

1 stalk celery, cut into
    small dice

2 medium-size carrots,
    peeled, halved length-
    wise, and sliced thinly

2 (4-inch) pieces fresh
    lemongrass, smashed

1 (4-inch) piece fresh gin-
    ger, peeled and sliced
    into quarter-size rounds

1 red chile, seeded, or 1 tea-
    spoon red pepper flakes

1 piece star anise

8 cups water

¼ cup vegan vegetable-
    flavor broth powder, or
    2 vegan vegetable-
    flavor bouillon cubes

1 (15-ounce) can
    coconut milk

¼ cup water chestnuts

½ cup shiitake or wood
    ear mushrooms

¼ cup baby corn, cut
    into pieces

14 fresh snow pea pods,
    stemmed and halved

¼ cup bamboo shoots

½ cup broccoli florets

2 tablespoons Florida
    Crystals

2 tablespoons lime juice

1 tablespoon tamari

Salt and pepper

Thinly sliced scallions,
    for garnish

Chopped fresh cilantro,
    for garnish

Note: You'll need to have cheesecloth on hand to make this recipe.

1. In a 6-quart stockpot over medium heat, sauté the onions, garlic, celery, and carrots in the sesame oil for 3 to 5 minutes, until slightly softened.

2. Put the lemongrass, ginger, chile, and star anise in a 12-inch square of cheesecloth and tie shut. Place in the pot.

3. Add the water, broth powder, and coconut milk to the pot and simmer over medium-low heat for 15 minutes.

4. Add the water chestnuts, mushrooms, baby corn, snow pea pods, bamboo shoots, and broccoli florets, and cook over low heat for another 15 minutes. Add the Florida Crystals, lime juice, and tamari.

5. Remove the cheesecloth packet, pressing the liquid into the pot.

6. Add salt and pepper to taste.

**TO SERVE: SPRINKLE WITH
SCALLIONS AND CHOPPED CILANTRO.**

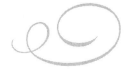

Salads

Many people think that salad is all that vegetarians eat. Salad is a great part of any diet—it's a chance to add fresh, crunchy vegetables to your meal and be creative with dressings and extra ingredients. Try adding the Baked Tempeh or Maple-Miso Dressing to your greens; add some kick to any salad with the crisp, cheeselike Tofu Nuggets. With its smoky tofu, sweet and savory dressing, toasted peanuts, and snow pea sprouts, our Gado Gado is one salad that'll quickly become a favorite of yours as well for lunch or dinner.

Salad can be a culinary adventure! Check out the produce aisle at your grocery store, or search your local farmers' market for tempting and inspiring elements. Don't limit yourself to produce—venture into grains and beans for extra taste and texture. These recipes should inspire you to be inventive.

Maple-Miso Dressing

Yield: 2 cups

*Sweet and salty, this dressing is
highly popular and oh-so-simple.*

¼ medium-size red onion,
  chopped coarsely
1 clove garlic
1 tablespoon miso
¾ cup maple syrup
¼ teaspoon ground ginger
1 cup extra-virgin olive oil
¼ cup tamari
½ cup water

1. Process all the ingredients in a blender until smooth.
Will keep in the refrigerator, tightly covered, for 3 weeks.

Tangy Tahini Dressing

Yield: 1½ cups

*Who says calcium is hard to come by for vegans? Certainly not if
you make this fabulous dressing a staple. Make only what you
need because this dressing is meant to be used within 2 days.*

½ cup tahini
1¼ cups water
2 tablespoons tamari
1 clove garlic
2 tablespoons chopped
  onion
¼ teaspoon dried basil
¼ teaspoon dried oregano
¼ teaspoon dried dill
¼ teaspoon ground cumin
¼ teaspoon black pepper
¾ teaspoon rice syrup
1 tablespoon fresh lemon
  juice
1½ tablespoons fresh
  minced parsley

1. Process all the ingredients in blender until smooth.

CHEF'S TIP: POUR LEFTOVER DRESSING OVER
LAYERED VEGETABLES AND BAKE, COVERED,
AT 350°F FOR 45 MINUTES FOR A DELICIOUS,
EASY CASSEROLE.

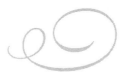

Fennel–Apple Dressing

Yield: 2 cups

This light, refreshing dressing is a delight on any salad.

4 dates, soaked in water
    for 1 hour
⅓ cup chopped cilantro
1 clove garlic
¼ teaspoon fennel seeds
1½ cups apple juice
1 tablespoon fresh
    lemon juice
1½ teaspoons grated ginger
1 scallion, chopped
Pinch of sea salt
¼ cup extra-virgin olive oil

1. Process all the ingredients in a blender until smooth.
Will keep for 4 days refrigerated.

Avocado Ranch Dressing

Yield: 2 cups

This thick, creamy dressing is our raw version of zesty ranch.
Avocado gives it body and makes it a perfect dipping sauce for
asparagus or steamed artichoke leaves. Romaine is a great lettuce
for this dressing as it supports its creamy texture well.

1½ medium-size Haas
    avocados, peeled
    and pitted
1 teaspoon minced garlic
2 tablespoons minced
    white onion
¼ cup fresh lemon juice
1½ tablespoons nama
    shoyu
1 teaspoon umeboshi
    plum vinegar
¼ cup extra-virgin olive oil
6 tablespoons nutritional
    yeast flakes
3 tablespoons agave syrup
½ cup water
Freshly ground pepper

1. Process all the ingredients in a blender until smooth.
Will keep for 3 days refrigerated.

Spicy French Dressing

Yield: 1 cup

This dressing has a little kick. With sweet, sour, and spicy flavors, this makes a great salad dressing or a dipping sauce for roasted potatoes or steamed vegetables.

¼ cup ketchup
¼ teaspoon hot sauce
¼ cup apple cider vinegar
4 teaspoons agave syrup
2 tablespoons extra-virgin olive oil
1 teaspoon brown rice miso
¼ cup minced celery
½ teaspoon minced garlic
2 tablespoons water
3 tablespoons canola oil

1. Process all the ingredients in a blender until smooth.

Will keep for up to 10 days refrigerated.

Smoky Toasted Sesame Dressing

Yield: 1¾ cups

This dressing is a basic Asian-style dressing with a tiny bit of smoky flavor.

½ cup canola oil
3 tablespoons toasted sesame oil
¼ cup apple cider vinegar
3 tablespoons wheat-free tamari
1 tablespoon agave syrup
2 tablespoons toasted sesame seeds

1. Whisk all the ingredients together.

Will keep for up to 2 weeks refrigerated.

Fresh Herb Vinaigrette

Yield: ¾ cup

This dressing is simple, light, and tart—perfect for brightening the flavor of your favorite salad greens. Try substituting any fresh herb you like, such as dill or sage.

½ teaspoon fresh thyme
½ teaspoon fresh oregano
¼ teaspoon fresh rosemary
1 tablespoon chopped fresh basil
¼ cup champagne vinegar
2 teaspoons Dijon mustard
½ teaspoon sea salt
½ cup extra-virgin olive oil
Freshly ground pepper

1. Finely chop all the herbs together.

2. Whisk in the vinegar, mustard, and salt. Slowly whisk in the olive oil and finish with freshly ground pepper to taste.

Will keep for 1 week refrigerated.

Croutons

Yield: 4 cups

1 loaf vegan Italian bread, cut into ½-inch cubes

3 tablespoons extra-virgin olive oil

½ teaspoon sea salt

½ teaspoon paprika

¼ teaspoon garlic powder

½ teaspoon Italian seasoning (see Spice Blends, page 23)

Preheat the oven to 350°F.

1. In a large bowl, toss the bread with the oil, salt, and paprika until each cube is coated.

2. Spread cubes in a single layer on a baking sheet. Bake for 6 to 7 minutes, turning often, until crisp.

Stored in an airtight container, these keep well.

Carrot-Tahini Slaw

Serves 6–8

This great summer salad is light and easy to prepare.

10 carrots, peeled and grated

1 small red onion, diced finely

3 stalks celery, peeled and diced

½ cup tahini

3 teaspoons tamari

Juice of 1 lemon

½ teaspoon sea salt

1 teaspoon dried dill

1 teaspoon Spike

½ cup toasted sunflower seeds

1. Combine all the ingredients except the sunflower seeds in a large bowl and mix well.

2. Cover and chill for an hour. Mix in the sunflower seeds and serve.

CHEF'S TIP: FILL AND ROLL A CABBAGE OR ROMAINE LEAF WITH THE CARROT MIXTURE FOR A TASTY HANDHELD LUNCH.

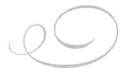

Salads

Chickpea Untuna Salad

Serves 4–6

1½ cups cooked chickpeas, or 1 (15-ounce) can, drained and rinsed

2 tablespoons minced red onion

1 stalk celery, finely diced

1 medium-size carrot, peeled and grated

¼ cup Vegenaise

¼ teaspoon dulse flakes

1 tablespoon nutritional yeast

¼ teaspoon dried oregano

1 teaspoon finely chopped fresh parsley, or 2 teaspoons dried

1 teaspoon chopped scallions

¾ teaspoon tamari

Pinch of black pepper

We really don't like to pretend that vegetables are meat or fish, but the dulse flakes in this salad add a delicious sea flavor, and the chickpeas are a good source of protein. This is so simple to make, you can have it around all the time for a pleasing sandwich filling.

1. In a mixing bowl, mash the chickpeas with a fork, then add the remaining ingredients and mix until incorporated.

To serve: Serve as a sandwich, a salad, or on toast points.

CHEF'S TIP: IF YOU FIND THE RED ONIONS ARE TOO STRONG FOR YOUR LIKING, RINSE THEM IN COLD WATER BEFORE USING.

Coleslaw

Yield: 6 cups; serves 6–8

1 head cabbage

¼ cup thinly sliced scallion

¼ cup grated carrot

3 stalks finely chopped celery

2 tablespoons finely chopped fresh parsley, or ½ teaspoon dried

½ cup Vegenaise

¼ teaspoon minced garlic

1½ teaspoons Florida Crystals

1 teaspoon Spike seasoning

⅛ teaspoon celery seeds

Salt and pepper

Everyone should have a good slaw recipe. This basic one can be jazzed up with creative variations such as toasted nuts and seeds, or some red bell pepper for a sweet and colorful addition. If you like a kick, spice it up with a shot of hot sauce.

1. Finely shred one-half of the cabbage, and grate the other half.

2. In a mixing bowl, toss all the ingredients together. Season to taste with salt and pepper.

CHEF'S TIPS: THE VEGENAISE AND SPIKE BRING OUT THE SAVORY FLAVOR.

The more salt you add, the more water will be brought out of the cabbage. For crispier slaw, add no salt.

VARIATION: FOR ADDED CRUNCH, ADD ½ CUP OF TOASTED SUNFLOWER SEEDS.

83

Dark Green Salad

Serves 6–8

Add or substitute any of your favorite seasonal vegetables or greens to make this the season's harvest in a bowl. As this salad marinates, it gets better and better.

4 cups dark greens (such as kale or collards), washed, chiffonaded (see Chef's Tip), and tightly packed

2 medium-size tomatoes, cut into medium dice

1 clove garlic, minced finely

½ medium-size summer squash, cut into small dice

½ cup shredded red cabbage

½ cup shredded green cabbage

½ cup shredded carrot

½ cup extra-virgin olive oil

Pinch of cayenne

½ teaspoon sea salt

2 tablespoons chopped sun-dried tomatoes

¼ cup apple cider vinegar

1 tablespoon agave syrup

½ cup broccoli florets, chopped finely

3 tablespoons raw sunflower or pumpkin seeds

1. In a large mixing bowl, combine all the ingredients and toss well to coat everything with the oil and vinegar. Let sit for 15 to 20 minutes to marinate.

CHEF'S TIP: TO CHIFFONADE
ANY KIND OF LEAFY GREENS,
REMOVE ANY TOUGH, THICK STALKS,
AND STACK THE LEAVES ACROSS EACH OTHER.
ROLL UP THE LEAVES TIGHTLY INTO A CIGAR SHAPE,
THEN SLICE THINLY ACROSS TO
CREATE STRIPS.

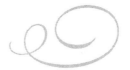

Eggless Tofu Salad

Serves 4–6

1 (14-ounce) block firm
   tofu, drained
½ cup Vegenaise
¼ cup celery, chopped finely
½ cup shredded carrots
2 tablespoons chopped
   fresh parsley, or
   ½ teaspoon dried
2 tablespoons stone-
   ground mustard
1 teaspoon onion powder
½ teaspoon sea salt
½ teaspoon garlic powder
½ teaspoon black pepper
½ teaspoon paprika
½ teaspoon turmeric
¼ cup nutritional yeast
1 tablespoon tamari

The possibilities are endless when it comes to using tofu. This take on a traditional salad is easy to prepare: everything goes into one bowl, and with a few pantry staple spices and a wave of your measuring spoons, you can create this addictive salad. Serve on a bed of greens with vegetables and crackers, or use as a sandwich filling.

1. Mash the tofu in a large bowl, then add all the remaining ingredients, blending well.

Soba Noodles in Peanut Sauce

Serves 4

8 ounces soba noodles
½ cup Peanut Sauce (page
   59)
¼ cup matchstick-cut
   carrots
¼ cup thinly sliced scallions
1 tablespoon toasted
   sesame oil
Pinch of sea salt
Sesame seeds, for garnish
Bean sprouts, for garnish

Savory and simple, these soba noodles are tossed in spicy peanut sauce and served with fresh carrots and scallions. Top with snow pea shoots and sesame seeds for a gourmet touch.

1. Fill a 6-quart stockpot with water and bring to a boil. Add the soba noodles to the boiling water and cook for 7 minutes.

2. Drain the noodles into a colander and run under cool water until slightly cool to the touch.

3. Using a medium-size bowl, toss together the noodles, peanut sauce, carrot, scallion, sesame oil, and a pinch of salt.

4. Serve family style or divide into individual servings, garnished with sesame seeds and sprouts.

Gado Gado

Serves 4

Many people who have tried this version of the Indonesian classic would say that gado gado means "more more" or "yum yum"! Crisp romaine lettuce, garden vegetables, smoky tofu strips, toasted peanuts, and snow pea shoots topped with our addictive Gado Gado dressing satisfies on many levels and makes a delicious meal.

1 (14-ounce) block firm tofu, cut into french-fry-size sticks

Gado Tofu Marinade
1½ teaspoons liquid smoke flavoring
¼ cup extra-virgin olive oil
2 tablespoons tamari

Gado Gado Dressing
¾ cup natural peanut butter
¼ cup chopped fresh cilantro
¼ teaspoon red pepper flakes
2¼ teaspoons tamarind pulp
6 tablespoons tamari
¼ cup water
¼ cup canola oil
Pinch of ground ginger
½ cup brown rice vinegar
¼ cup maple syrup
1 clove garlic
2¼ teaspoons Florida Crystals

Salad
1 head romaine lettuce, torn into bite-size pieces
6 ounces prewashed mesclun mix
¼ cup shredded green cabbage
¼ cup shredded red cabbage
¼ cup shredded carrot
2 tablespoons chopped roasted peanuts
½ teaspoon toasted sesame seeds
2 scallions, chopped
Snow pea shoots, for garnish (optional)

Make the Gado Tofu Marinade:

Preheat the oven to 350°F.

1. Mix the Gado Tofu Marinade ingredients together.

2. Line a baking sheet with baking parchment, then brush the parchment with the marinade. Arrange the strips of tofu evenly on the baking sheet and brush the tops with the marinade.

3. Bake for 20 minutes, or until puffed up.

Make the Gado Gado Dressing:

1. Blend all the ingredients in a blender until smooth.

Assemble the Salad:

1. In a large bowl, toss together the romaine and mesclun. Divide among four plates, and evenly portion out the cabbage, carrot, and peanuts.

2. Place strips of smoky baked tofu on each plate and drizzle each salad lightly with the dressing.

3. Sprinkle with the sesame seeds and scallions. For a more festive garnish, top with a bundle of spring pea shoots.

Greek Salad

Serves 6

One bite of this salad of marinated, fetalike tofu cheese, crisp romaine lettuce, sun-dried tomatoes, and Greek olives will take you to the Mediterranean.

1 (14-ounce) block firm tofu, rinsed and patted dry

Dressing
2 tablespoons red wine vinegar

2 tablespoons fresh lemon juice

3 tablespoons extra-virgin olive oil

½ teaspoon dried basil

½ teaspoon dried oregano

1 teaspoon sea salt

2 teaspoons umeboshi paste

½ teaspoon freshly ground black pepper

Salad
1 medium-size cucumber, peeled and seeded

¼ cup Greek olives

½ red onion, chopped

1 head romaine lettuce, torn into bite-size pieces

1 ripe tomato

2 tablespoons marinated sun-dried tomatoes, minced

1. Crumble the tofu into a medium-size mixing bowl.

Make the Dressing:
1. In a separate bowl, mix together the dressing ingredients, whisk well, and pour over the crumbled tofu. Cover the bowl with plastic wrap and refrigerate to allow the tofu to marinate (overnight for best flavor).

Assemble the Salad:
1. Slice the cucumber in half lengthwise, cut into half-moons, and add to the bowl of marinated tofu. Add the olives and red onion, and toss with the tofu and dressing.

2. Just before serving, place the romaine in a large salad bowl and add a scoop of the tofu mixture. Cut the tomato in half, slice thinly, and garnish the salad. Serve at once.

Quinoa Salad

Serves 4–6

Quinoa, a complete protein, was an ancient superfood used by the Aztecs. Make this power food a staple in your family's pantry.

3 cups water

½ teaspoon sea salt

2 cups quinoa, rinsed well and drained

½ medium-size red onion, diced

1 large carrot, grated

1 medium-size red bell pepper, diced

1 cup fresh or thawed frozen corn kernels

Dressing

¼ cup fresh lemon juice

2 tablespoons extra-virgin olive oil

½ cup finely chopped cilantro

2 cloves garlic, minced

1 teaspoon sea salt

½ teaspoon black pepper

Make the Quinoa:

1. In a medium-size saucepan over high heat, bring 3 cups of water and the salt to a boil and add the quinoa.

2. When the water returns to a boil, turn the heat down to a simmer, cover, and cook for 20 minutes, or until all the water is absorbed. Remove from the heat and let rest for 10 minutes, covered.

3. Transfer the quinoa into a medium-size bowl and set aside.

Make the Dressing:

1. Combine the lemon juice, oil, cilantro, garlic, salt, and pepper in a mixing bowl and whisk well.

Assemble the Salad:

1. Add the onion, carrots, red pepper, and corn to the quinoa, pour in the dressing, and mix well.

2. Refrigerate for 30 minutes to allow the quinoa to absorb the flavors.

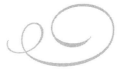 CHEF'S TIP: QUINOA IS A WONDERFULLY TASTY AND NUTRITIOUS GRAIN, BUT IT COMES WITH A BITTER COATING CALLED SAPONIN THAT MUST BE RINSED OFF BEFORE COOKING.

Sea Caesar/
Cruelty-Free Caesar

Serves 4

Light and refreshing, Sea Caesar derives its name from the inclusion of nori and Hijiki Caviar. Cruelty-Free Caesar has the tangy flavor of black olives and sun-dried tomatoes. Whichever you choose makes a fantastic starter or a tasty meal with the addition of baked tofu or tempeh croutons.

Make the Caesar Dressing:

1. In a blender, process all the dressing ingredients except the oils and salt. With the blender running, add the oils slowly to emulsify. Add salt to taste.

Make the Salad Base:

1. Toss the romaine with the cabbage, carrots, and dressing in a large salad bowl.

Assemble the Sea Caesar:

1. Top each serving with ¼ cup Hijiki Caviar, a sprinkle of nori strips, a bit of diced celery, and some scallions.

Assemble the Cruelty-Free Caesar:

1. Toss the salad with chopped olives and sun-dried tomatoes, and sprinkle each serving with croutons and Sprinkle "Cheese."

Caesar Dressing

¼ cup lemon juice

1 clove garlic

½ tablespoon capers

1 tablespoon prepared mustard

1½ teaspoons nutritional yeast

1¼ teaspoons black pepper

1 teaspoon tamari

½ cup extra-virgin olive oil

½ cup canola oil

Sea salt

Salad Base

4 hearts of romaine, washed and chopped or torn into bite-size pieces

¼ cup carrot, cut into matchsticks

¼ cup shredded green cabbage

¼ cup shredded red cabbage

To Assemble Sea Caesar

1 sheet nori, toasted and cut into thin strips

1 cup Hijiki Caviar (recipe follows)

¼ cup diced celery

Thinly sliced scallion, for garnish

To Assemble Cruelty-Free Caesar

8 black olives, chopped

8 sun-dried tomatoes, chopped

Croutons, for garnish

¼ cup Sprinkle "Cheese" (page 60)

Hijiki Caviar

Yield: 4 cups

This can be enjoyed warm or cold and is
delicious served on toast points.

1 cup dried hijiki

3 cups warm water, for
soaking

2 tablespoons untoasted
sesame oil

2 small onions, cut into
small dice

4 cloves garlic, minced

1 tablespoon minced fresh
ginger

1 scallion, minced

1 tablespoon brown rice
vinegar

3 tablespoons mirin

3 tablespoons lemon juice

¼ cup tamari

1 tablespoon toasted
sesame oil

1 tablespoon agave syrup

Pinch of cayenne

Salt and pepper

1. In a large bowl, soak the hijiki in warm water for 15 minutes.

2. Heat the oil in a large skillet over low heat. Add the onion, garlic, ginger, and scallion, and sauté for 5 to 7 minutes.

3. Stir in the hijiki and cook for 2 minutes more.

4. Increase the heat to medium, add the brown rice vinegar, mirin, and lemon juice, and cook for 2 to 3 minutes.

5. Add the tamari, toasted sesame oil, agave syrup, and cayenne and stir to coat.

6. Remove from the heat and season with salt and pepper.

Spinach Salad with Baked Beets, Spiced Pecans, and Balsamic Dressing

Serves 6

8 ounces baby spinach,
washed well

Baked Beets

4 medium-size beets,
trimmed and halved

3 tablespoons extra-virgin
olive oil

Sea salt

Beets are at their peak of freshness in the summer, so take full advantage of their sweet flavor. This salad is filled with beautiful gems. It looks gorgeous plated; add some pomegranate seeds for a mine full of rubies. The caramelized nuts are great to keep around as a sweet treat for any salad.

Bake the Beets:

1. Bring a 4- to 6-quart pot of salted water to a boil, add the beets, and boil for 15 to 20 minutes, until slightly soft.

2. Preheat the oven to 400°F. Line a baking sheet with baking parchment.

3. Drain and rinse the beets in cold water and remove their skin under cool water.

4. Chop the beets into bite-size pieces and toss in a medium-size bowl with the oil. Spread on the prepared baking sheet. Bake for 20 minutes.

5. Remove the beets from the oven. Sprinkle lightly with salt. Set aside to cool.

Make the Dressing:

1. Whisk together the oil, vinegar, salt, and pepper. Add the garlic and let sit in the dressing until time to dress the salad.

Make the Spiced Pecans:

1. Toast the pecans in a dry sauté pan for 5 minutes. Remove from the pan and set aside.

2. Combine the maple syrup, oil, and tamari in a sauté pan and heat until bubbling. Cook for 3 to 5 minutes, until sticky. Add the cinnamon, cayenne, and pecans, and toss to coat the nuts. Transfer the nuts to a sheet of baking parchment. When cool, separate and chop roughly.

Assemble the Salad:

1. In a large mixing bowl, lightly dress the spinach with the Balsamic Dressing.

2. Divide the spinach among the plates, scatter the roasted beets on top, and sprinkle the spiced pecans around the edge of the salad.

Balsamic Dressing

¼ cup extra-virgin olive oil

2 tablespoons balsamic vinegar

Salt and pepper

1 clove garlic, smashed

Spiced Pecans

½ cup pecans

2 tablespoons maple syrup

1 tablespoon grape seed, sunflower, or other flavorless oil

1 teaspoon tamari

¼ teaspoon ground cinnamon

Pinch of cayenne

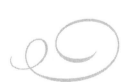

Tofu Nuggets

Serves 4–6

These B$_{12}$-rich nuggets are crispy and cheeselike morsels of baked tofu. People who try these become instant fans, and the nuggets are a special hit with kids. Serve hot or cold as a tasty snack or atop a salad.

2 (14-ounce) blocks firm tofu, drained and cut into 1-inch cubes

½ cup extra-virgin olive oil, plus 2 tablespoons for coating pan

1 tablespoon tamari

¾ cup nutritional yeast

1 tablespoon dried thyme

1 tablespoon Spike

Preheat the oven to 450°F. Line a baking sheet with baking parchment, and coat the parchment with 2 tablespoons of the oil.

1. Place the cubed tofu in a medium-size bowl and pour the remaining ½ cup of oil and tamari over it; toss to coat. Sprinkle the dry ingredients over the tofu and toss again.

2. Spread the tofu cubes on the prepared sheet and bake for 20 to 25 minutes, turning once during the baking process to ensure even browning.

Roasted Tomato, Basil, and Corn Salad

Yield: 5 cups; serves 4

3 large tomatoes, cut into medium dice

½ small red onion, cut into small dice

¼ teaspoon red pepper flakes, or a pinch of cayenne

2 tablespoons extra-virgin olive oil

2–3 grinds freshly ground black pepper

1 teaspoon sea salt

4 ears fresh corn, or 3 cups canned or frozen corn

½ cup fresh basil leaves, torn into small pieces

1 tablespoon minced fresh parsley

1 tablespoon balsamic vinegar

Sea salt

Preheat the oven to 425°F. Line a baking sheet with baking parchment.

1. In a bowl, combine the tomatoes, onions, red pepper flakes, olive oil, pepper, and salt. Mix well, and spread out on the prepared baking sheet. Roast for 20 minutes, turning halfway through the baking process.

2. While the tomatoes are roasting, take the corn off the ears, if using fresh corn, and combine with the basil and garlic.

3. Add the corn to the mixture on the hot baking sheet and return to the oven for another 5 minutes. Remove from the oven and let everything cool down for about 10 minutes.

4. Add the basil, parsley, and balsamic vinegar. Refrigerate and serve chilled.

Tara's Mediterranean
Pasta Salad

Serves 6–8

1 pound pasta of choice (I like brown rice elbows)

⅓ cup olive oil

6 large cloves garlic, minced

1 medium-size onion, diced

½ cup black olives, sliced

15 green olives (with or without pimiento), sliced

¼ cup capers, drained

1 pound frozen sliced tricolored peppers

1 tablespoon Italian seasoning (see Spice Blends, page 23)

10 marinated artichoke hearts, diced

The truth is that this recipe, created by our friend Tara, was invented due to laziness. According to Tara, "I had planned to cook pasta for dinner and realized that I was out of tomato sauce. Since I did not feel like making a trip to the grocery, I opted to make do with items I had stored in my refrigerator and pantry.

Perhaps it would be more appropriate to name the recipe Tara's Lazy Mediterranean Pasta Salad!"

1. Cook the pasta according to package directions, rinse with cool water, and set aside.

2. Warm the olive oil over medium heat. Add the garlic and onion, and sauté for 2 to 3 minutes. Add the Italian seasoning. Add the frozen peppers, stirring until the color is vibrant and peppers are almost warm.

3. Turn down the heat and add the remaining ingredients except for the artichoke hearts. Sauté for another 2 to 4 minutes, or until the peppers are warm. Be careful not to overcook the peppers—they should retain their bright color.

4. Toss together the pasta and sauce in a large bowl. Add the artichoke hearts. Serve hot or cold.

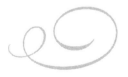

CHEF'S TIP: FOR SIMPLE VARIATIONS,
ADD ANY LEFTOVER STIR-FRIED VEGGIES (BROCCOLI,
CARROTS, CAULIFLOWER, ZUCCHINI, OR YELLOW SQUASH)
DURING STEP 3. A 15-OUNCE CAN OF DICED TOMATOES
ALSO MAKES A NICE ADDITION.

Sandwiches and Wraps

Sandwiches and wraps are some of the easiest and most satisfying meals for people on the go. The recipes here feature vegan renditions of old favorites, as well as exciting new flavor combinations. The Wheatball Sub transforms the classic Italian meatball sub into a hearty, healthy lunch. The Philly Seitan Sandwich is all-out decadence with its deliciously cheesy flavors and delectable sautéed greens, and our classic Club Sandwich features the savory flavors of baked tofu, Tempeh Bacon, and Veganaise on toasted whole-grain bread. The real showstopper is the Earth Burger, a blend of pantry staples that creates one of the best meatless burgers you'll ever have.

BBQ Tofu Wrap

Serves 6

2 (14-ounce) blocks extra-firm tofu, drained and cut lengthwise into 6 pieces

1 cup Barbecue Sauce (recipe follows), plus extra reserved for topping

2 tablespoons extra-virgin olive oil

6 whole wheat tortillas

1 medium-size red onion, sliced thinly

2 large tomatoes, sliced thinly

6 romaine lettuce leaves, sliced thinly

Pepper

VARIATION: ADD ONE-QUARTER OF A SLICED AVOCADO TO EACH WRAP FOR EXTRA TASTE AND NUTRITION.

Use this spicy, sweet barbecue sauce to either grill or bake the tofu for this wrap. Fill it with shredded carrots, romaine lettuce, and diced tomato. Served with corn on the cob, coleslaw, and potato salad, this makes a perfect picnic treat.

1. Put the tofu slices on a baking sheet. Mix the barbecue sauce with the oil and brush half the mixture onto the slices. Flip the slices and brush with the remaining sauce. Cover and marinate for at least 1 hour, or overnight for extra-tender tofu.

2. Preheat the grill and grill the tofu on each side for 5 minutes, or until seared. Or preheat the oven to 350°F, and bake the tofu on a baking parchment–lined baking sheet for 7 to 10 minutes on each side, until lightly browned.

3. To assemble a wrap, place a tortilla on your work surface. Place two slices of the tofu in the center of the tortilla; top with lettuce, tomato, red onion, and additional barbecue sauce; sprinkle with pepper.

4. Fold in the sides of the tortilla and roll firmly from the bottom to the top. Slice each wrap in half on the diagonal. Repeat with remaining tortillas and serve.

Sandwiches and Wraps

Barbecue Sauce

Yield: 3 cups

This spicy sauce will keep well, tightly covered in the refrigerator, for 2 to 3 weeks, or frozen for up to 2 months.

3 whole dried ancho chiles, seeded and stemmed

1½ teaspoons extra-virgin olive oil

2 cups diced onions

7 cloves garlic

1 cup tomato paste

½ cup vegetarian Worcestershire sauce

⅓ cup brown sugar

¼ cup apple cider vinegar

¼ cup lemon juice

4½ tablespoons mustard

2 teaspoons sea salt

1. Rehydrate the chiles in hot water for 10 minutes, or until soft.

2. In a skillet, sauté the onions and garlic in the olive oil until soft, and add the drained chiles.

3. In a blender or food processor, process the chile mixture with the remaining ingredients until smooth.

CHEF'S TIP: FOR A SPICIER SAUCE,
USE CHIPOTLES PACKED IN ADOBO SAUCE,
AND SKIP THE REHYDRATING STEP.

Broccoli-Seitan Knishes

Yield: 12 knishes

In this new take on a traditional Jewish classic, we add seitan, broccoli, and onions to make a hearty treat. This is a good way to use up last night's cold mashed potatoes. Try using other vegetables, such as spinach and/or mashed yams, for the filling. These are a great lunch with a cup of soup or salad and can be frozen.

4 large potatoes, peeled and cut into pieces

4 cups water

1 medium-size onion, chopped finely

8 cloves garlic, chopped finely

8 ounces seitan, drained and sliced thinly

¼ cup extra-virgin olive oil

1 cup chopped broccoli

2 teaspoons sea salt

2 tablespoons tamari

1 teaspoon turmeric

1 teaspoon black pepper

1 teaspoon dried thyme

1 teaspoon Spike

2½ cups unbleached all-purpose flour

2 teaspoons baking powder

¼ cup potato cooking water, plus more as needed

1. Cook the potatoes in the boiling water in a medium-size pot for 25 minutes, or until tender. Drain, reserving the cooking water. Set aside.

2. Sauté the onion, garlic, and seitan in the olive oil in a skillet over medium heat for 5 to 10 minutes. Add the broccoli and cook for 2 minutes more.

3. Mash the potatoes. Stir half of the mashed potatoes into the broccoli mixture. Season with ½ teaspoon of the sea salt and 1 tablespoon of the tamari.

CHEF'S TIP:
THE DOUGH MAY BE
ROLLED OUT TO FORM
LARGER SQUARES
AS NEEDED TO
ACCOMMODATE FILLING.

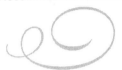

4. Preheat the oven to 375°F. Line a baking sheet with baking parchment.

5. Mix the remaining potatoes with the turmeric, the remaining 1½ teaspoons of the sea salt, and the pepper, thyme, Spike, flour, and baking powder to create a dough. Add ¼ cup of the potato water and knead. Add more potato water as needed until dough is soft and comes together.

6. Turn out the dough onto a floured surface and knead for a few minutes. Roll out into a ¼-inch-thick rectangle and cut into twelve 4-inch squares.

7. Scoop ½ cup of filling onto the middle of each of the squares. Bringing the opposite corners together, fold the dough over the filling, and pinch closed to form a pouch.

8. Place the pouches seam side down on the lined baking sheet. Brush the tops with oil and bake for 20 to 25 minutes, until golden brown.

Club Sandwich

Serves 1

3 slices whole wheat bread

Vegenaise

2 slices Baked Tofu (page 53)

3 slices Tempeh Bacon (page 37)

2 slices tomato

2 leaves lettuce

This mouthwatering version of a country club favorite will get you into any club you desire. Smoky tempeh and baked tofu pair up to make this an all-time favorite.

1. Lightly toast the bread. Spread each slice with Vegenaise to taste.

2. On the bottom slice, lay one or two pieces of tofu and, on top of that, three tempeh bacon strips.

3. Cover with the middle slice of bread, and layer on the tomato, then the lettuce.

4. Cover with the last slice of bread and slice diagonally into two or four triangles, using toothpicks to keep the layers together.

Earth Burger

Yield: 12 burgers

1 (14-ounce) block
    firm tofu, pressed
    (see Chef's Tip)

1 tablespoon extra-virgin
    olive oil, plus extra for
    brushing

1 tablespoon canola oil

1 medium-size onion,
    chopped finely

2 cloves garlic,
    chopped finely

1 cup finely chopped
    carrots

1 cup quick-cooking oats

1½ cups sunflower seeds

2 cups cooked brown rice

1 tablespoon chopped
    fresh parsley

1 tablespoon Spike

1 tablespoon white miso

1 tablespoon lemon juice

1 tablespoon dried thyme

1 tablespoon dried basil

3 tablespoons tamari

¾ cup bread crumbs

6 tablespoons water

Oil, for brushing

Pantry staples come together to create the best burger on this planet. A blend of tofu, brown rice, oats, sunflower seeds, vegetables, and spices, this is a crowd-pleaser. Even though it makes a big batch, it won't make it to the freezer.

Preheat the oven to 350°F. Oil and then line a baking sheet with baking parchment.

1. In a large bowl, mash the tofu thoroughly and set aside.

2. In a medium-size pan, sauté the onion, garlic, and carrots in the teaspoon of olive oil and the canola oil over medium heat until soft but not brown. Transfer to the bowl with the mashed tofu.

3. Add to the tofu mixture all the remaining ingredients except the water and the oil reserved for brushing.

4. Process in batches in a food processor until everything is well blended, adding the water a tablespoon at a time until the mixture binds together.

5. Form into ½-cup burgers.

6. Place the burgers on the prepared baking sheet and bake for 20 minutes, turning the baking sheet halfway through the baking process to ensure even browning.

After cooking, these burgers can be frozen in an airtight container for up to 2 months. Thaw fully before reheating.

CHEF'S TIP: TO PRESS TOFU, PLACE A BLOCK OF TOFU
BETWEEN TWO PLATES. PLACE A HEAVY OBJECT (SUCH AS
A CAN OR TWO OF BEANS) ON TOP OF THE TOP PLATE
AND LET SIT FOR A HALF HOUR. POUR OFF THE
WATER AND PAT THE TOFU DRY.

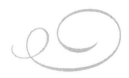

Philly Seitan Sandwich

Yield: 4 sandwiches

2 (12-inch) loaves
  Italian bread

4 cups thinly sliced seitan

¼ cup tamari

3 tablespoons extra-virgin
  olive oil

½ cup Caramelized Onions
  (page 55)

Nutro Cheese (page 59)

Sautéed Greens (page 65)

Roasted red peppers,
  sliced thinly

East Coast flavor in a bun. We have transformed this Philly-style sandwich into a vegan version made even more scrumptious with thinly sliced seitan and caramelized onions, to which we've added calcium-rich sautéed greens and B vitamin–rich nutritional yeast cheese. Serve these with Cajun-Spiced Baked Potato Fries (page 63) for all-out decadence.

Preheat the oven to 350°F. Line a baking sheet with baking parchment.

1. Toss the sliced seitan with the tamari and olive oil. Spread out on the prepared baking sheet and bake for 6 to 8 minutes, or until golden.

2. Slice the loaves in half lengthwise and place in the oven a minute or two to warm.

3. Mix the seitan and caramelized onions together and spread out on the split loaves.

4. Smother with the Nutro Cheese. Fold the bread over the filling and cut each loaf in half to create four sandwiches. Serve with sautéed greens and roasted red peppers.

Sandwiches and Wraps

Falafel

Yield: 12 falafel; serves 2

All the traditional flavors of the Middle East, wrapped in freshly made flatbread. Serve accompanied by Tahini Sauce and vegan herbed Cucumber Salad.

½ cup bulgur

½ teaspoon extra-virgin olive oil, plus extra for baking

1 cup cooked chickpeas, or one (15-ounce) can, drained and rinsed

½ large onion, cut into small dice

1 tablespoon chopped fresh parsley, or 1 teaspoon dry

1 tablespoon ground flaxseeds

2 cloves garlic

½ teaspoon salt

1 teaspoon red pepper flakes

1 teaspoon ground cumin

⅛ teaspoon dried coriander

Tahini Sauce (recipe follows)

2 whole wheat pita breads, halved

Shredded lettuce, for serving

Sliced tomato, for serving

Preheat the oven to 350°F. Coat a large baking sheet with olive oil.

1. Soak the bulgur in warm water to cover for at least ½ hour.

2. Sauté half the onion in 1 teaspoon of the olive oil until slightly soft.

3. Combine the chickpeas, all the onion, and the parsley, flaxseeds, garlic, salt, and spices in a food processor and blend until combined but not totally smooth.

4. Drain the bulgur and stir enough into the chickpea mixture so that the latter is no longer sticky. Form the falafel mixture into golf ball–size balls and flatten slightly. Place, well spaced, on the oiled baking sheet.

5. Bake for about 15 minutes or until golden brown, turning the sheet around halfway through the baking time.

6. Serve in the warm pita halves with shredded lettuce, diced tomato, and tahini sauce.

Tahini Sauce

Yield: ¾ cup

¼ cup tahini

6 tablespoons water

1 teaspoon fresh lemon juice

2 cloves garlic, minced

Pinch of sea salt

1. Combine all the sauce ingredients in a blender and blend until smooth.

Cucumber Salad

Serves 4

2 cups plain soy yogurt
¼ cup minced fresh mint
  leaves
2 tablespoons lemon juice
2 small cloves garlic,
  minced
2 pinches white pepper
2 medium-size cucumbers,
  peeled, seeded, and
  chopped
Sea salt

1. Mix all the ingredients and chill.

Gyros

Serves 4

This sandwich takes some time to prepare, but you'll find it is well worth the effort when you wrap your mouth around these juicy layers of seitan with zesty Moroccan-style marinade in homemade bread or whole wheat pita filled with crisp romaine and tomatoes dressed with a creamy, cool cucumber sauce.

Cucumber Dressing
1 (12.3-ounce) package
  firm silken Lite Tofu,
  drained and crumbled
½ cup peeled and finely
  chopped cucumber
1 tablespoon extra-virgin
  olive oil
2 teaspoons fresh lemon
  juice
¼ teaspoon sea salt
¼ teaspoon black pepper

Moroccan Marinade
1 cup tomato juice
⅓ cup fresh orange juice
⅓ cup fresh lemon juice
2 tablespoons tamari
3 cloves garlic
2 tablespoons rice syrup
⅓ teaspoon red pepper
  flakes
⅔ teaspoon ground
  coriander

**Make the
Cucumber Dressing:**

1. Put the tofu, cucumber, olive oil, lemon juice, salt, and pepper in a blender or food processor and process to form a chunky sauce. Set aside.

**Make the
Moroccan Marinade:**

1. In a small bowl, combine the marinade ingredients and whisk together.

103

⅛ teaspoon ground
  cinnamon

⅛ teaspoon ground cumin

⅔ teaspoon ground
  fennel seeds

1¼ teaspoons minced
  fresh ginger

1½ teaspoons balsamic
  vinegar

Sandwiches

Canola oil, for frying

2 cups seitan, thinly sliced

Gyro Bread (recipe fol-
  lows) or 4 whole wheat
  pita breads

2 cups bite-size pieces
  romaine lettuce

1 tomato, seeded and
  chopped

1 small red onion, sliced
  thinly

Make the Sandwiches:

1. Coat a skillet with a thin layer of canola oil over medium heat. When hot, lay the seitan slices in the pan in a single layer and brown on both sides.

2. Pour the marinade into the skillet over the browned tofu and cook for 3 to 5 minutes. Remove from the heat and set aside.

3. Place the breads on a clean surface and divide the seitan equally among them. Top the seitan with the lettuce, tomato, and onion, then the dressing.

4. Fold over the bread and eat taco style.

Gyro Bread

Yield: 4–6 loaves

2¼ cups warm water,
  approximately 104°F

1 tablespoon active
  dry yeast

1 tablespoon Sucanat

3 tablespoons extra-virgin
  olive oil

1½ teaspoons sea salt

3 cups unbleached
  pastry flour

Preheat the oven to 400°F.

1. In a medium-size bowl, combine the water, yeast, and Sucanat. Let sit in warm spot for 5 minutes, until foamy.

2. Mix in 1 tablespoon of the olive oil and the salt. Add the flour slowly until the dough comes together—it should be soft but not too sticky.

3. Turn out the dough onto a lightly floured surface and knead for10 minutes, until smooth and elastic.

4. Coat the inside of a clean bowl with the remaining 2 tablespoons of the olive oil and place the dough inside; roll the dough around in the oiled bowl to coat all surfaces.

5. Cover the dough with plastic wrap and let rise for 20 to 30 minutes, until doubled in size.

6. Lightly knead the dough and divide into four to six balls. Roll out each piece into a thin rectangle approximately 5 by 7 inches. Poke all over with a fork, place on a baking sheet, and bake for 3 to 5 minutes.

The bread can be reheated by putting it in a 200°F oven for 3 to 4 minutes.

If you don't have the time to make the bread, you can easily substitute pita.

CHEF'S TIPS:
WRAP THE HOT BREAD IN FOIL TO KEEP IT PLIABLE UNTIL SERVING.

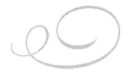

Quinoa-Avocado Wrap with Orange Baked Tofu

Yield: 6 wraps

The combination of quinoa, tofu, and avocado provides your body with all the essential fats and protein needed to keep it healthy and satisfied. Fill these with any of your favorite vegetables to create a nutritious, flavorful, and satisfying lunch.

Tofu Marinade

1 cup orange juice

½ cup lemon juice

¼ cup brown rice syrup or maple syrup

½ cup chopped fresh cilantro

1 teaspoon extra-virgin olive oil

½ teaspoon sea salt

1 (14-ounce) block extra-firm tofu, cut into ¼-inch slices

Wraps

2 cups cooked quinoa

3 ripe avocados, peeled, pitted, and sliced

2 large tomatoes, sliced thinly

1 medium-size onion, sliced thinly

1 medium-size cucumber, peeled, seeded, and sliced thinly

6 large whole wheat tortillas

Make the Tofu Marinade:

1. Put the orange juice, lemon juice, rice syrup, cilantro, cumin, salt, and olive oil in a blender and mix until well combined.

2. Place the tofu slabs in a single layer in a shallow baking dish and pour the tofu mixture over the top. Cover and let marinate for 30 to 60 minutes.

3. Preheat the oven to 375°F and bake the tofu on a baking parchment–lined baking sheet for 18 minutes.

Assemble the Wraps:

1. Place a tortilla on your work surface.

2. For each wrap, put ⅓ cup of quinoa in the center of the tortilla and top with an avocado half, tomato, onion, and cucumber. Cut one slab of tofu per wrap into strips and scatter on top.

3. Fold in both sides of the tortilla and roll tightly from the bottom to the top. Repeat with the other tortillas. Slice each wrap in half on the diagonal and serve.

Italian-Style Tofu Cutlet Sandwich

Serves 6

1 medium-size yellow onion, diced

4 cloves garlic

2 tablespoons extra-virgin olive oil

2 tablespoons Italian seasoning (page 23)

2 (14-ounce) blocks firm tofu

1 teaspoon minced fresh parsley

1 teaspoon sea salt

½ teaspoon pepper

2 tablespoons nutritional yeast

1 tablespoon garlic powder

3 tablespoons vegan vegetable-flavor broth powder, or 1 vegan vegetable-flavor bouillon cube, dissolved in 2 tablespoons hot water

¼ cup dry white wine, mirin, or water

1 tablespoon tamari

2 cups bread crumbs

6 rolls of your choice

1 cup vegan mozzarella, shredded

Sprinkle "Cheese" (page 60), for sprinkling

These flavor-filled patties are made by blending tofu with Italian spices, coating with bread crumbs, and baking. Serve these as a sandwich with sautéed greens or over pasta with marinara sauce for a delightful meal.

Preheat the oven to 375°F. Lightly oil a baking sheet and set aside.

1. Sauté the onions and garlic in the olive oil over medium heat until golden, then stir in the Italian seasoning.

2. Crumble the tofu into a medium-size mixing bowl, and add the parsley, salt, pepper, nutritional yeast, and garlic powder. Mix to incorporate everything. Add the sautéed onion and garlic to the tofu mixture.

3. Pour the reconstituted broth into the sauté pan. Raise the heat to medium and whisk the liquid to deglaze the pan. Add to the tofu mixture.

4. Transfer the tofu mixture to the bowl of a food processor and process, adding 1 cup of bread crumbs until the mixture comes together and is a bit sticky.

5. Pour the remaining cup of bread crumbs into a shallow pan. Portion the tofu mixture out into golf ball–size balls, flatten into patties, and coat each side with the bread crumbs. Place on the oiled baking sheet and bake for 12 minutes, or until golden.

6. Place one patty on a split roll, sprinkle with vegan mozzarella, and bake until the cheese is bubbly. Top with some Sprinkle "Cheese," fold each sandwich closed, and enjoy.

Wheatball Sub
(a.k.a. Wheatball Hoagie, Wheatball Grinder, Wheatball Hero)

Serves 4

1½ pounds seitan, about 5 cups

2 cups fresh bread crumbs, tightly packed

¼ cup extra-virgin olive oil, plus extra for brushing

2 medium-size onions, diced

6 cloves garlic, minced

1½ cups dry bread crumbs

1 cup tomato sauce

1 tablespoon Spike

1 tablespoon Italian seasoning (page 23)

1 tablespoon plus 1 teaspoon tamari

2 tablespoons dried basil

4½ teaspoons dried oregano

4½ teaspoons dried rosemary

2 submarine rolls

1½ cups House Marinara (page 58), for spooning over the rolls

Sautéed Greens (page 65)

Sprinkle "Cheese" (page 60), for sprinkling

This is a classic Italian meatball sub transformed with wheat, the classic American grain, into a healthful vegan lunchtime sandwich. For the pasta lover, these wheatballs can also be substituted into the traditional spaghetti and meatballs.

Preheat the oven to 350°F. Line a baking sheet with baking parchment.

1. In a food processor fitted with the metal blade, grind the seitan until crumbled finely. Add the fresh bread crumbs to the seitan.

2. In a large pan, warm the ¼ cup of olive oil over medium heat and add the onion and garlic. Sauté until soft, then add to the processer bowl containing the seitan mixture.

3. Add all the remaining ingredients, and process together in the food processor until a doughlike mixture comes together.

4. Scoop out ¼-cup measures of the mixture and roll into balls. Place the wheatballs on the prepared baking sheet and lightly oil the tops of the wheatballs. Bake for 15 minutes.

5. To assemble the sandwiches, place the wheatballs in a split sub roll with House Marinara, sautéed greens, and Sprinkle "Cheese."

Sandwiches and Wraps

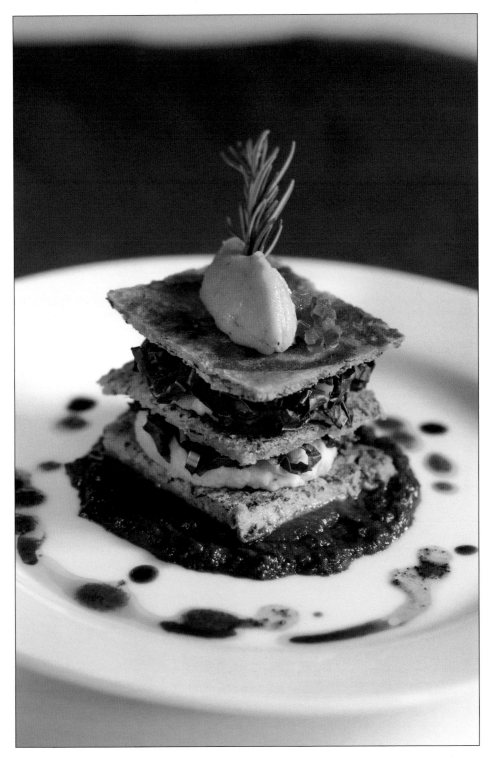

Chickpea Socca, recipe on page 130

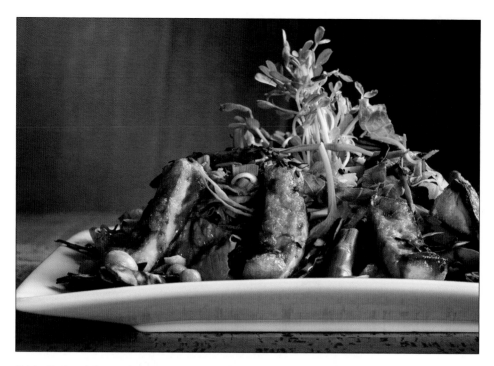

Gado Gado, recipe on page 86

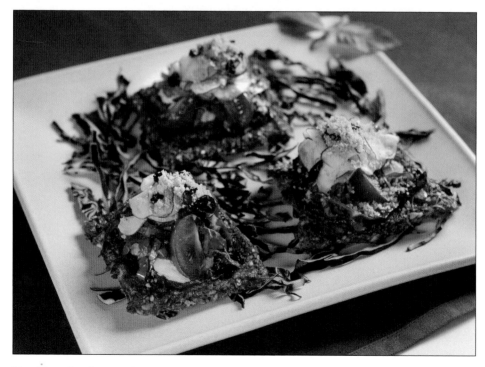

Live Pizza Crackers, recipe on page 157

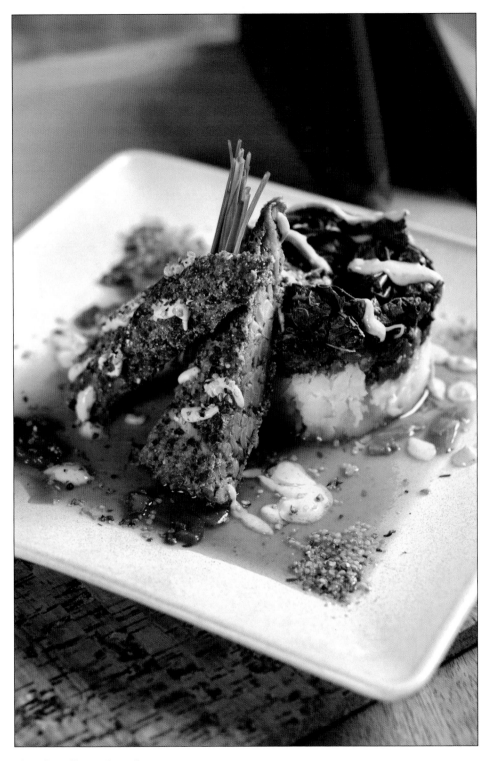

Blue Corn Hempeh, recipe on page 129

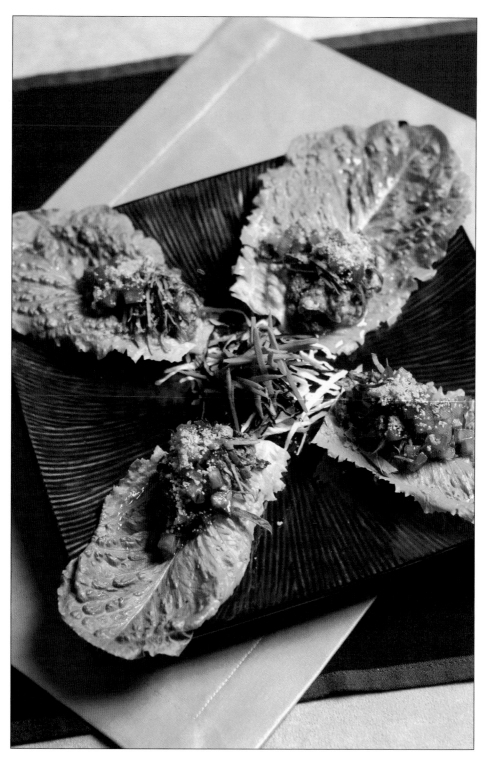

Leaf Wraps, recipe on page 152

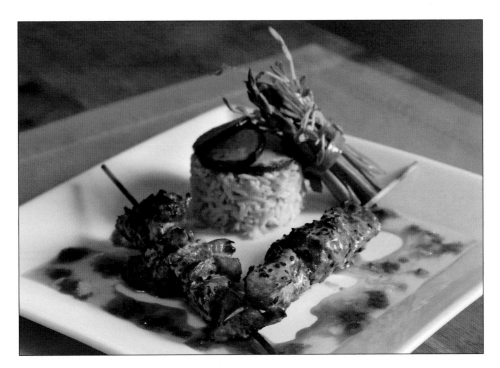

Seitan Satay, recipe on page 140

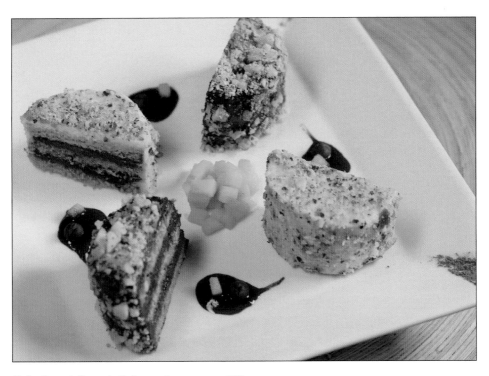

Rain Forest Crunch Cake, recipe on page 189

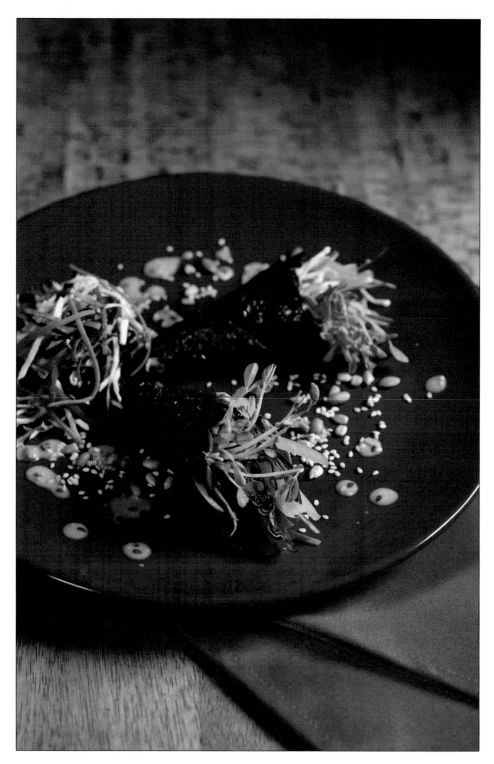

Raw Maki Hand Roll, recipe on page 161

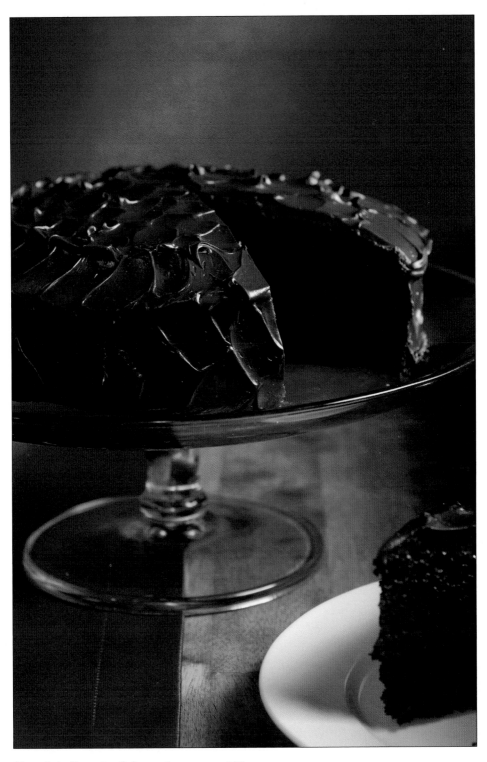

Chocolate Ganache Cake, recipe on page 185

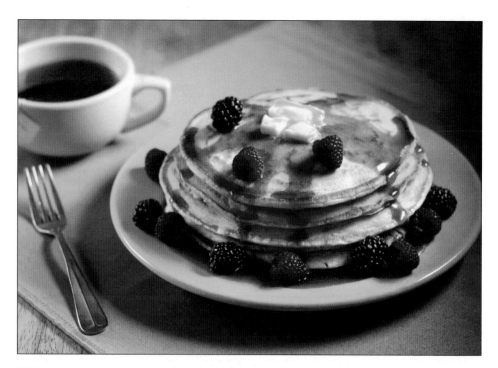

Tiffany's Pancakes, recipe on page 37

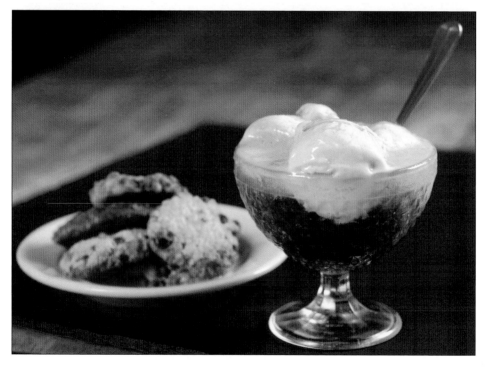

Magic Cookies and Root Beer Float, recipes on pages 173 and 44

Appetizers

As the introduction to a meal, appetizers tease and tantalize the palate with a hint of the dining experience that lies ahead. The following section offers creative adaptations of some of our favorite appetizers. You can serve these before a meal, or even as the main dish. The Collard Rolls are a great addition to any potluck, while our Marinated Stuffed Mushrooms with Tempeh Sausage and Garlic Aioli will have guests at an elegant cocktail party swooning. You won't find a better barbecue combo than the Potato Skins and Spicy Tofu Hot Wings. Silver dollar–size Zucchini-Pecan Pancakes with Spicy Maple Syrup are another savory summertime treat. No matter what you choose or how you serve them, these recipes offer a delicious variety of tempting flavors.

Collard Rolls Stuffed with Quinoa, Sweet Potato, and Caramelized Onions

Serves 6 as an appetizer, 4 as an entrée

This hearty appetizer takes full advantage of winter's bounty.
Emerald collards and a golden lentil sauce create a
rich feast of color for the eye. Packed with protein,
this dish also makes a satisfying entrée.

12 large or 24 small collard leaves, stalks removed

Sea salt

Minced fresh parsley, for garnish

Filling

2 teaspoons extra-virgin olive oil

½ large onion, cut into medium dice

1½ cups medium-dice sweet potato

1½ tablespoons minced garlic

½ cup quinoa, washed well and drained

1¼ cups vegan vegetable stock (page 52)

½ teaspoon dried basil

½ teaspoon dried oregano

1. Blanch the collard leaves in liberally salted boiling water for about 1 minute, then plunge into ice water. Reserve the cooking water.

Make the Filling:

1. In a 4- to 6-quart stockpot, heat the oil and sauté the onions until browned and slightly sticky. Add the diced sweet potato, garlic, and herbs, and sauté until soft (about 10 minutes). Add the quinoa and stock, and bring the mixture to a boil. Turn down the heat to simmer, cover, and cook for 20 minutes.

2. Preheat the oven to 350°F.

3. Lay out the collard leaves stalk side down and spoon 2 to 3 tablespoons of the cooked filling onto each leaf, leaving a margin to fold in along each side. Fold in both sides of the leaves and roll into bundles.

4. Place the rolls seam side down in a baking pan, and pour the reserved collard water into the bottom of the pan. Cover the pan with foil and bake for 20 minutes.

Appetizers

Lentil Sauce

2 teaspoons extra-virgin
   olive oil

½ large red onion,
   minced finely

1 clove garlic,
   minced finely

½ cup finely minced celery

2 cups vegan
   vegetable-flavor broth

½ cup lentils, rinsed
   and sorted

1 tablespoon fresh
   lemon juice

1½ teaspoons mirin or
   white wine

1 teaspoon tamari

1 tablespoon dried dill

1 teaspoon dried thyme

Salt and pepper

Make the Lentil Sauce:

1. In the meantime, heat a large saucepan over medium heat. Add the oil, onions, celery, and garlic, and sauté until softened. Add the broth, lentils, lemon juice, wine, tamari, dill, and thyme, and bring to a boil.

2. Turn down the heat to a simmer and cook for 15 minutes, or until the lentils are soft. Add salt and pepper to taste.

TO SERVE:
SPREAD THE LENTIL SAUCE
UNDER THE COLLARD ROLLS AND
SPRINKLE WITH FRESH PARSLEY.

Cornmeal Cakes with Pico de Gallo

Yield: 15 corn cakes

When fresh corn and tomatoes are at their peak, make these easy-to-prepare crispy golden cakes. Top them with our juicy Pico de Gallo and light tofu sour cream—your guests will think you spent hours over a hot stove.

Tofu Sour Cream (page 61)

Make the Pico de Gallo:

1. Place all the sauce ingredients in a bowl and mix well.

Pico de Gallo

1 large tomato, seeded and
   cut into fine dice

½ medium-size red onion,
   chopped finely

¼ cup finely chopped
   cilantro, washed well

2 jalapeños, seeded and
   chopped

1 teaspoon sea salt

Juice of ½ lemon

Corn Cakes

1 tablespoon baking powder

¼ teaspoon baking soda

1½ cups whole-grain cornmeal

1½ cups unbleached all-purpose flour

2½ cups soy milk

3 tablespoons soy margarine, melted

1 tablespoon vegan egg replacer

1½ tablespoons maple syrup

1 teaspoon sea salt

1½ cups corn kernels

Canola or other flavorless oil, for frying

Make the Corn Cakes:

1. In a medium-size bowl, mix together the baking powder, baking soda, cornmeal, and flour.

2. In a separate bowl, mix together the soy milk, melted margarine, egg replacer, maple syrup, and salt.

3. Add the wet ingredients to the dry and stir to incorporate. Add the corn kernels and mix well.

4. Heat a large skillet over medium heat until hot, then lightly brush with the oil.

5. Drop ¼ cup corn cake batter into the oil and fry on each side until golden brown, 2 to 3 minutes per side.

6. Transfer the corn cakes to plates. Top each corn cake with pico de gallo and a dollop of tofu sour cream.

Creamy Chickpea Hummus and Oatmeal–Garlic Crackers

Serves 4–6

Everyone loves hummus. Ours is a creamy blend of chickpeas, cumin, garlic, fresh lemon juice, and sea salt. It's easy and nutritious, and people will absolutely flip for these homemade crackers.

Preheat the oven to 350°F.

Oatmeal-Garlic Crackers

3 cups uncooked rolled oats

1½ cups sunflower seeds

¾ cup whole wheat pastry flour

1½ teaspoons garlic powder

1 teaspoon toasted and ground cumin

¾ teaspoon sea salt

½ cup melted coconut oil

½ cup brown rice syrup

6 tablespoons water

3 tablespoons mixed sesame, poppy, and caraway seeds, for topping

Make the Crackers:

1. In a food processor, separately grind the oats and sunflower seeds until fine and transfer to a large bowl.

2. Stir together the flour, garlic powder, and salt in a bowl, and mix into the oat mixture.

3. In a separate bowl, whisk together the coconut oil and rice syrup.

CHEF'S TIP: USING A RULER
TO GUIDE A PIZZA CUTTER
MAKES SCORING THESE
CRACKERS A QUICK AND
EASY JOB.

4. Add the wet ingredients to the dry, mixing in water as needed to produce a stiff yet pliable dough.

5. Roll out the dough between two sheets of baking parchment to just slightly greater than ⅛-inch thickness. Make sure the thickness is uniform throughout.

6. Remove the top sheet of parchment and score the dough all the way through into 2-inch squares, then across diagonally to create triangles. Slide the parchment onto a baking sheet.

7. Sprinkle the seed mixture liberally over the dough. Press in gently.

8. Bake until lightly browned, 15 to 20 minutes. (Crackers on the outer edges of the pan will brown more quickly than those near the center.) Remove from the oven and score again. Transfer to a wire rack and cool completely.

Make the Hummus:

1. In a food processor, blend all the hummus ingredients until smooth.

**TO SERVE: SERVE THE HUMMUS
ACCOMPANIED BY THESE
HOMEMADE CRACKERS AND/OR SOME
RAW VEGETABLE CRUDITÉS.**

Hummus

¼ cup extra-virgin olive oil

2 cloves garlic

Pinch of cayenne

½ teaspoon sea salt

4 teaspoons fresh lemon juice

2 cups cooked chickpeas

¼ cup water

¼ cup tahini

¾ teaspoon toasted and ground cumin seeds

Crispy Wonton Packages

Serves 8

Show off your international cooking skills with these bite-size crispy cocktail appetizers. Shredded cabbage, sweet sesame carrots, shiitake mushrooms, and sliced baked tofu–filled packages will go fast, but this recipe makes a lot. They may be prepared ahead and reheated before the party.

Wonton Filling

1 tablespoon extra-virgin olive oil

2 cloves garlic, minced

½ cup thinly sliced napa cabbage

3 scallions, sliced thinly

5 shiitake mushrooms, sliced thinly

5 fresh snow pea pods, trimmed, cleaned, and sliced thinly

¼ cup diced carrots

3 slices baked tofu (page 53) cut into ¼-inch cubes

½ teaspoon Sucanat

1 tablespoon tamari

1 teaspoon sesame oil

1 (12-ounce) package wonton wrappers

3 cups canola or other flavorless oil, for frying

Arrowroot Paste

1 teaspoon arrowroot

2 tablespoons water

Dipping Sauce

½ teaspoon tamari

¼ teaspoon minced fresh ginger

3 tablespoons rice vinegar

3 tablespoons peanut butter

2 tablespoons toasted sesame oil

2 tablespoons agave syrup

½ cup water

1 teaspoon white miso

Pinch of cayenne

Make the Wonton Filling:

1. Heat a large sauté pan over medium heat. When hot, pour the olive oil into the pan. Add the garlic and stir until slightly golden.

2. Add all the vegetables and sauté for 1 to 2 minutes. Add the tofu and stir to heat. Remove from the heat and set aside to cool. Mix in the Sucanat, tamari, and sesame oil.

Make the Arrowroot Paste:

1. Thoroughly stir the arrowroot powder into the water to make a paste.

Prepare the Dipping Sauce:

1. Whisk together all the sauce ingredients in a medium-size bowl, and set aside.

Make the Wontons:

1. In the center of each wonton wrapper, place a small mound of filling (about 1 teaspoon) and brush arrowroot paste around the edge. Fold each wrapper in half over the filling, and seal the wontons by pressing the edge with a fork.

2. In a deep skillet, heat the 3 cups of flavorless oil over high heat.

3. When the oil is hot, cook the wontons for 2 to 3 minutes on each side until golden brown. Transfer to paper towels to drain. Serve hot with the dipping sauce.

Appetizers

Grilled Zucchini Rollatini with Sun-Dried Tomatoes and Olives

Serves 8

2 large zucchini, sliced thinly lengthwise
2 tablespoons balsamic vinegar
¼ cup canola oil
6 tablespoons Dijon mustard
2 cloves garlic
2 tablespoons tamari
2 tablespoons fresh lemon juice
Freshly ground black pepper
Dash of hot sauce
¼ cup Tofu Cheese (page 60)
3 tablespoons chopped sun-dried tomatoes
1 tablespoon chopped black olives
Fresh herbs, for garnish

People will gobble up these tasty and pretty appetizers at any gathering. The mix of the smoky grilled zucchini, tangy tofu cheese, sweet and salty tomatoes, and olives will keep their lips smacking.

Preheat a grill or broiler with a rack arranged 3 inches from the heat.

1. Process the vinegar, oil, mustard, garlic, tamari, lemon juice, pepper, and hot sauce in a blender until well mixed.

2. Brush the mixture on the zucchini slices and let marinate for 15 to 20 minutes.

3. Grill the zucchini slices until soft and pliable.

4. Mix the tofu cheese with the sun-dried tomatoes and chopped black olives. Put a dollop of tofu cheese mixture on one end of each zucchini strip and roll up. Sprinkle with herbs to serve.

CHEF'S TIP: STICK A SPRIG OF FRESH ROSEMARY
IN EACH ONE AND SPRINKLE WITH MINCED PARSLEY
FOR A BRIGHT, BEAUTIFUL DISPLAY.

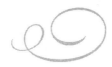

Marinated Stuffed Mushrooms with Tempeh Sausage and Garlic Aioli

Serves 8

Perfect as a pass-around appetizer at the table of your most elegant affair. This versatile delight is easy to prepare but hard to pass up. The creamy garlic aioli also makes a delicious spread for sandwiches, especially with toasted focaccia.

Aioli

1½ cups Vegenaise

2 tablespoons lemon juice

3 tablespoons extra-virgin olive oil

1 tablespoon stone-ground mustard

Pinch of cayenne

2 cloves garlic, minced

¼ teaspoon sea salt

Chopped fresh parsley, for garnish

Mushrooms

24 medium-size mushrooms, cleaned and stemmed

¼ cup balsamic vinegar

½ cup extra-virgin olive oil

¼ cup tamari

Sausage Filling

8 ounces Marinated Tempeh (page 55)

¼ cup fresh bread crumbs

2 tablespoons extra-virgin olive oil

2 tablespoons tamari

Pinch of dried marjoram

¼ teaspoon dried thyme

¼ teaspoon paprika

Pinch of cayenne

¼ teaspoon fennel seeds

Pinch of black pepper

2 tablespoons unbleached all-purpose flour

Preheat the oven to 400°F.

Make the Aioli:

1. Whisk together the Vegenaise, oil, mustard, lemon juice, garlic, cayenne, and salt. Chill in the refrigerator until cool.

Make the Mushrooms:

1. Mix the oil, vinegar, and tamari in a medium-size bowl. Toss the mushrooms in the mixture to lightly coat. Let sit 10 minutes, then arrange the mushrooms on a baking sheet, hollow side up.

Make the Sausage Filling:

1. While the mushrooms are resting, crumble the tempeh into a bowl. Add the bread crumbs, herbs, oil, tamari, and flour. Mix well.

2. Spread the mixture on a baking sheet and bake for 10 to 15 minutes, until slightly crumbly. Remove from the oven and let cool.

3. Fill the mushrooms with the tempeh sausage and place in the oven for 10 to 15 minutes.

4. Sprinkle the stuffed mushrooms with the parsley. Arrange on a serving platter and drizzle with the aioli.

Pan-Grilled Mushroom Tapenade

Serves 6–8

This rich and smoky mix of mushrooms, olives, and onions makes a robust topping for crisp baguette with a thin layer of the light parsley-infused Tofu Cheese. Try any favorite combination of mushrooms you would like or change the olives for different flavors.

Toast Points

12 slices of baguette, sliced as thinly as possible (ideally ⅛-inch thick)

2 tablespoons extra-virgin olive oil

Pinch paprika

Tapenade

¼ medium-size yellow onion, chopped

1 tablespoon extra-virgin olive oil

1 tablespoon water

2 large portobello mushrooms, sliced

3 medium-size shiitake mushrooms, sliced

1 teaspoon tamari

1 teaspoon liquid smoke flavoring

¼ cup minced green olives

1 scallion, minced

2 tablespoons minced fresh parsley, for garnish

Make the Toast Points:

Preheat the oven to 350°F.

1. In a large bowl, toss the baguette slices in the olive oil and paprika until coated.

2. Spread out on a baking sheet and bake for 6 minutes, or until golden.

Make the Tapenade:

1. In a skillet over medium heat, cook the onion, oil, and water for approximately 2 minutes. Add the mushrooms and cook for 2 minutes more. Add the liquid smoke and tamari, and cook until everything is caramelized.

2. Remove from the heat and add the chopped olives, scallions, and parsley. Serve warm or at room temperature on the toast points.

TO SERVE:
PREPARE TOFU CHEESE (PAGE 60)
AND SPREAD THINLY ON TOAST
BEFORE TOPPING WITH MUSHROOMS.

Potato Skins

Serves 6 as an appetizer, 2 as an entrée

Crispy baked potato skins filled with creamy tofu sour cream, zesty salsa, and smoky tempeh bits. Top with our tasty Three-Bean Chili to make it a delicious meal.

3 large potatoes, rinsed

1 tablespoon extra-virgin olive oil

1 teaspoon paprika

Pinch of sea salt

1 cup Three-Bean Chili (page 73)

1 cup Live Salsa (page 156)

½ cup Tofu Sour Cream (page 61)

Preheat the oven to 350°F. Line a baking sheet with baking parchment.

1. Fill a large stockpot with salted water and bring to a boil. Add the whole potatoes and cook for 20 minutes, or until they can be easily pierced with a knife, but the skins are not splitting.

2. Drain and cover the potatoes with cold water for 10 minutes. Remove the potatoes from the water, cut in half lengthwise, and gently scoop out the insides with a spoon, leaving a sturdy shell.

3. Place the potato halves on the prepared baking sheet, skin side down. Drizzle the halves with olive oil and sprinkle with the paprika and sea salt. Bake for 20 to 25 minutes, or until golden.

4. Fill with the chili and top with the salsa and sour cream.

CHEF'S TIP: THESE POTATO SKINS CAN BE TOPPED WITH ANY FILLING YOU LIKE, SUCH AS GUACAMOLE, BLACK BEANS, OR CHUTNEY.

What to Do with the Insides of Your Potato Skins:

When you make potato skins, you will have leftover cooked potato from their insides. Here are some of the many things you can do with this valuable part of the potato. If you don't have time to use the insides of the potatoes right away, they can be refrigerated and used the next day.

Mashed potatoes: If the potato is not soft enough to mash, place back in the pot, covered with water, and boil for 4 to 5 minutes. Drain, then mash with a little soy milk, olive oil, and salt and pepper.

Oven-baked home fries: Preheat the oven to 400°F, toss the potato pieces with 1 teaspoon of olive oil, ½ teaspoon of garlic powder, and ¼ teaspoon of paprika, and salt and pepper to taste, then bake until browned.

Use for Potato-Leek Soup (page 72) or **Broccoli-Seitan Knishes** (page 98).

Radiance's Fried Polenta Appetizer

Yield: 20 balls; serves 4–5

This heirloom recipe has been served for over thirty years in our friend Radiance's family, and she is very excited to share it with the world.

3½ cups water

¼ tablespoon sea salt

1 cup cornmeal

1 tablespoon fresh chopped parsley, or 1 teaspoon dried

1½ teaspoons fresh chopped oregano, or ½ teaspoon dried

1 cup House Marinara (page 58)

1½ cups canola or other flavorless oil

1. Bring the water to a boil in a large, heavy kettle. Add the salt.

2. Turn down the heat to a simmer and add the cornmeal in a steady stream, stirring all the while. Continue to cook and stir for 20 minutes after all the cornmeal has been added. The polenta is done once it pulls away from the sides of the pot.

3. Remove from the heat and stir in the fresh herbs. Allow the polenta to cool for 5 minutes, then scoop it into your hands with a teaspoon and form into balls.

4. Heat the oil in a deep, heavy pan until hot and fry the balls in batches, so that they are not crowded in the pan, until golden brown. Drain on paper towels.

Serve with the House Marinara for dipping.

Scallion Pancakes with Plum and Dipping Sauces

Yield: 12 pancakes, to make 6 pancake sandwiches

Fill these crispy pancakes with smoky Tempeh Bacon and plum sauce for an exotic treat. The fermented black beans can be found at an Asian food store and are worth the trip.

Plum Sauce

1 cup plum preserves

½ cup fermented black beans

1 cup water

1 ¼-inch piece fresh ginger, peeled and minced

2½ small cloves garlic

¼ cup Sucanat

½ teaspoon sea salt

Make the Plum Sauce:

1. Puree all the plum sauce ingredients in a blender until smooth.

2. Transfer the mixture to a saucepan and cook over low heat for 10 to 15 minutes, or until thick and spreadable.

Scallion Pancakes

4 cups unbleached
  all-purpose flour

1 cup sesame oil

½ teaspoon sea salt

¼ cup sesame seeds

¼ cup sliced scallions

2 tablespoons canola or
  other flavorless oil, for
  brushing pancakes

Dipping Sauce

2 tablespoons Sucanat

2 tablespoons tamari

⅛ teaspoon wasabi powder

4 teaspoons toasted
  sesame oil

½ teaspoon Spike

2 tablespoons water

½ teaspoon minced
  fresh ginger

1 piece star anise

1 scallion, minced

Make the Scallion Pancakes:

1. In a mixing bowl, mix together the flour, salt, and sesame oil until crumbly.

2. Slowly add the water a little bit at a time and stir until the dough comes together and is pliable but not sticky.

3. Divide the dough into twelve balls and roll each in the sesame seeds and scallions. Flatten into pancakes with a rolling pin, pressing in the seeds and scallions.

4. Heat a skillet over medium heat and brush the pancakes with the flavorless oil. Fry the pancakes for 2 to 3 minutes per each side until golden brown. Keep the finished pancakes warm and covered in a 200°F oven until ready to eat.

Make the Dipping Sauce:

1. In a blender, blend all the dipping sauce ingredients except for the scallions, then strain out any solids. Stir in the minced scallions.

TO SERVE: SPREAD THE PLUM SAUCE
BETWEEN TWO PANCAKES AND
SERVE WITH THE DIPPING SAUCE.

Tofu Hot Wings

Serves 4–6

No vegan potluck is complete without this spicy take on the finger-food classic. The hot sauce was created by our fiery friend Maegan. Be sure to make plenty—these wings will surely fly!

Hot Wing Sauce

¼ medium-size red onion,
  chopped roughly

2 cloves garlic, chopped

½ cup extra-virgin olive oil

1 tablespoon lime juice

2 tablespoons hot sauce

1 tablespoon Dijon mustard

2 tablespoons Vegenaise

2 tablespoons water

¼ cup rice vinegar

½ tablespoon sea salt

Pinch of black pepper

½ teaspoon agave nectar
  (optional)

Make the Hot Wing Sauce:

1. Sauté the onion and garlic in 2 tablespoons of the olive oil over medium heat until slightly browned at the edges.

2. Transfer to a blender and add the lime juice, hot sauce, mustard, Vegenaise, water, vinegar, salt, and pepper. Blend. With machine running, slowly add the remaining 6 tablespoons of olive oil.

3. If desired, add ½ teaspoon of agave nectar. Set aside.

Cool Ranch Dressing

½ clove garlic

2 tablespoons roughly
   chopped white onion

2 stalks celery with leaves,
   chopped

4 ounces tofu, crumbled

1 tablespoon cider vinegar

⅓ cup Vegenaise

½ teaspoon Spike

1 tablespoon fresh
   lemon juice

⅛ teaspoon black pepper

Pinch of cayenne

⅓ cup unsweetened
   soy milk

¼ cup extra-virgin olive oil

Tofu Wings

1 (14-ounce) block
   firm tofu

⅔ cup canola or other
   flavorless oil

Dredging Mixture

⅓ cup unbleached
   all-purpose flour

1 teaspoon garlic powder

1 teaspoon paprika

1 teaspoon sea salt

1 teaspoon pepper

Make the
Cool Ranch Dressing:

1. Process all the ingredients except the olive oil in a blender until smooth. With the blender running, slowly blend in the olive oil. Set aside.

Make the
Tofu Hot Wings:

1. Slice the tofu block in half lengthwise, then cut each half into seven sticks.

2. Over medium-high heat, heat the oil in a 9-inch skillet.

3. Sift the dredging ingredients into a mixing bowl and toss the tofu gently in the mixture to coat. Shake off excess flour and place into hot oil.

4. Cook until the tofu puffs and crisps, carefully flipping the tofu over with a spatula halfway through the cooking process. Remove the tofu from the pan and drain on paper towels.

5. Toss the tofu in the Hot Sauce to coat.

**TO SERVE: SERVE WITH SMALL BOWLS OF
ADDITIONAL HOT SAUCE AND COOL
RANCH DRESSING AND SOME CELERY STICKS.**

Tortilla Torte with Creamy Pumpkin-Seed Pesto

Serves 8

This tasty layered torte is filled with sun-dried tomatoes, tofu cheese, olives, sautéed portobello mushrooms, and spinach. The bright green pesto is a zippy addition and is also great to use as a topping for a myriad of things from pasta to our golden home fries or mashed potatoes.

Spring mesclun mix, for serving

Tortilla Filling
10 cloves garlic, peeled

1 tablespoon plus 1 teaspoon extra-virgin olive oil

2 large portobello mushroom caps, sliced into strips

½ pound baby spinach, washed well

2 tablespoons water

3 (9-inch) whole wheat tortillas

½ cup Tofu Cheese (page 60)

½ cup chopped sun-dried tomatoes

¼ cup sun-dried black olives

2 tablespoons nutritional yeast

Pesto Dressing
¼ cup toasted pumpkin seeds

1 cup chopped stemmed fresh parsley

1 cup fresh basil, tightly packed

2 cloves garlic

5 tablespoons extra-virgin olive oil

1 tablespoon water

2 teaspoons miso

2 tablespoons nutritional yeast

Preheat the oven to 350°F. Oil a baking sheet or line it with baking parchment.

Make the Filling:

1. Sprinkle the garlic cloves with 1 teaspoon of the olive oil and a pinch of salt, and wrap in a piece of foil. Bake for 20 minutes, then remove from the oven and allow to cool. When cool, mince.

2. In a sauté pan, cook the portobello caps in the remaining teaspoon of olive oil until soft. Add the spinach and 2 tablespoons of water, and continue cooking until the spinach is wilted.

3. Lay one tortilla on the prepared baking sheet. Spread with one layer of Tofu Cheese and sprinkle with half of the sun-dried tomatoes, olives, spinach, and portobellos.

4. Layer on a second tortilla and repeat the previous step.

5. Set the last tortilla on top and brush liberally with olive oil. Sprinkle with the nutritional yeast and bake for 15 minutes.

Prepare the Pesto:

1. While the tortilla bakes, prepare the pesto. Toast the pumpkin seeds on a dry baking sheet in the oven for 8 minutes, until puffed. Remove from the oven and set aside to cool.

2. In a blender or food processor, blend the parsley, basil, garlic, in and olive oil until puréed. Add the cooled

pumpkin seeds and process until smooth, then add the water, miso, and nutritional yeast, adding more water or oil to reach a spreadable consistency.

To Assemble:

1. When the tortilla is done, remove from the oven and slice into eight wedges. Serve over the mixed spring greens and drizzle with the pesto sauce.

Zucchini-Pecan Mini Pancakes

Yield: 12 pancakes; serves 4–6

These tasty zucchini-packed cakes are a great way to get the non-vegetable-eaters in your life to eat their vegetables. Pecans lend sweetness and add another level of texture to the pancakes. The spicy maple pecan sauce is also delicious on sautéed greens or any vegetables, and will keep well when refrigerated.

Spicy Maple Sauce

½ cup extra-virgin olive oil

½ small onion, chopped finely

3 cloves garlic, minced

1 cup maple syrup

2 teaspoons sea salt

¼ teaspoon cayenne

½ cup finely chopped toasted pecans

Make the Spicy Maple Sauce:

1. In a sauté pan over medium heat, heat the oil and sauté the onions and garlic until soft. Turn down the heat to medium-low and stir in the maple syrup, salt, and cayenne. Cook for 2 minutes.

2. Transfer the mixture to a blender and process until smooth. Mix in the toasted pecans and allow to cool.

Zucchini Pancakes

1 cup soy milk

1 medium-size zucchini,
 ends trimmed, grated

¼ cup canola oil

½ medium-size onion,
 diced finely

1 cup unbleached
 all-purpose flour

1 teaspoon baking powder

1 teaspoon baking soda

1 teaspoon sea salt

½ cup chopped pecans

¼ cup extra-virgin
 olive oil, for frying

Make the Zucchini Pancakes:

1. Combine the soy milk, grated zucchini, chopped onion, canola oil, and salt in a bowl.

2. In a separate bowl, stir together the flour, baking powder, baking soda, and pecans.

3. Add the dry mixture to the wet and mix well.

4. Heat 1 tablespoon of olive oil in a large skillet over medium heat.

5. Pour ¼ cup of the batter into the pan and cook until the top bubbles and the bottom is golden. Flip the pancake and cook the other side for 3 to 4 minutes. Repeat with the remaining batter, adding more oil if needed. Serve hot with the Spicy Maple Sauce.

Appetizers

Entrées

Like traditional meat-based dishes, these entrées form the centerpiece of a meal, with an array of starters and desserts playing supporting roles. Some of these recipes take a little longer to prepare, but you'll find they're worth the effort. These main courses are created with wholesome ingredients such as grains and beans, and such traditional soy foods as miso, tofu, and tempeh. A delectable introduction to tempeh is our Blue Corn Hempeh. Another high-protein staple we use is seitan, an especially popular meat alternative made from the gluten in wheat. Our Seitan Satay uses Thai-influenced flavors for a dish that makes even the most die-hard meat-eaters hungry for more.

For an extra gourmet meal, try the Wild Rice Risotto Cakes or our Chickpea Socca—a more formal, wheat-free adaptation of the traditional Mediterranean street food. Even confirmed carnivores will love these inventive, dazzling dishes.

Blue Corn Hempeh

Serves 4

This dish is a great introduction to eating tempeh. The marinated tempeh is coated with hempseeds, cornmeal, and crunchy blue corn chips, then topped off with a zesty mustard sauce. It's accompanied by mashed potatoes, mushroom gravy, sautéed greens, and a Southern classic, tomato pudding, all stacked into a comfort-food tower.

8 ounces Marinated Tempeh (page 55), cut in half lengthwise

¾ cup canola or other flavorless oil

Tomato Pudding (recipe follows)

Mushroom Gravy (page 58)

Sautéed Greens (page 65)

Yellow Mustard Sauce

¼ cup olive oil

1 medium-size onion, chopped

5 cloves garlic, minced

½ teaspoon paprika

½ teaspoon turmeric

¼ teaspoon sea salt

1 tablespoon drained capers

¼ cup prepared yellow mustard

⅓ cup water

½ (12.3-ounce) box silken lite tofu

Dredging Mixtures

2 cups crushed blue corn tortilla chips

½ cup hempseeds

½ cup unbleached all-purpose flour

1 cup whole-grain cornmeal

1½ teaspoons paprika

1 teaspoon dried thyme

1 cup unsweetened soy milk

2 tablespoons Dijon mustard

Make the Yellow Mustard Sauce:

1. Sauté the onion and garlic in the oil. When the onion is translucent, add the paprika, turmeric, and sea salt, and continue to sauté until the onions are soft.

2. Place the onion mixture in a blender with the remaining sauce ingredients and blend until smooth.

Make the Dredging Mixtures:

1. Process the corn chips and hempseeds in a food processor until finely ground. Add the remaining dredging ingredients, except the soy milk and mustard. Set the hempeh coating aside in a bowl or on a baking sheet.

2. Whisk together the soy milk and mustard, and set aside in a shallow bowl.

Make the Tempeh:

1. Dredge the tempeh slices first in the soy milk mixture, shaking off the excess, then in the hempeh mixture, coating completely.

2. In a large skillet, heat the canola oil over medium-high heat to 350°F, or until a small piece of hempeh coating dropped into the oil floats to the top and bubbles.

3. Fry the tempeh slices until golden and crispy, turning over halfway through the frying process. Drain on paper towels.

4. Serve with the yellow mustard sauce, accompanied by tomato pudding, mashed potatoes and mushroom gravy, and sautéed greens.

Entrées

Tomato Pudding

Serves 6

This is a vegan version of a Southern classic. We use it as a component to the Blue Corn Hempeh, but it is sweet and fabulous on its own.

1 (26-ounce) can diced tomatoes

2 cups cubed vegan bread

¼ cup coconut oil or vegan margarine

¼ cup molasses

¼ cup Sucanat

1 tablespoon extra-virgin olive oil

1 teaspoon sea salt

2 pinches black pepper

Preheat the oven to 375°F.

1. Mix together all the ingredients.

2. Pour the mixture into an ungreased 9 by 13-inch baking dish and bake for 45 minutes, or until the edges are brown and bubbling.

Chickpea Socca

Serves 4

We've elevated this traditional Mediterranean street food to a more formal and healthier level. Served with delicious sautéed dark greens and garlicky white beans, this wheat-free dish is satisfying and nutritious.

House Marinara (page 58)

Sautéed Greens (page 65)

White Bean Puree

2 cups cooked white beans, or 1 (15-ounce) can, drained and rinsed

½ cup minced fresh parsley

6 cloves garlic, roasted

3 tablespoons extra-virgin olive oil, or as needed

¼ teaspoon sea salt, or to taste

Caramelized Leeks

2 teaspoons extra-virgin olive oil

2 medium-size leeks, well washed and sliced thinly

½ teaspoon sea salt

Make the White Bean Puree:

1. In a blender or food processor, blend together the beans, parsley, and garlic. Add enough oil to achieve a rich and creamy consistency. Add sea salt to taste.

Make the Caramelized Leeks:

1. Heat the oil in a sauté pan over medium-low heat.

2. Add the leeks and the salt, and cook, stirring often, until the leeks begin to caramelize and turn a golden brown, 10 to 15 minutes. Remove from the heat and set aside.

Make the Socca:

Socca

2 cups chickpea flour

½ teaspoon sea salt

2 tablespoons herbes de Provence (page 24)

3 cups warm water

½ cup extra-virgin olive oil

1. Combine the chickpea flour, salt, and herbs in a medium-size bowl. Add the water and whisk until smooth. Whisk in the oil, cover, and allow to rest 1 hour.

2. Preheat the oven to 450°F. Oil a 9 by 13-inch baking dish and heat in the oven for 2 minutes.

3. Take the pan out of the oven, rewhisk the batter, and pour it into the hot pan.

4. Return the pan to the oven and bake for 18 to 25 minutes, until the socca is set and starts to crisp.

5. Remove the pan from the oven and score the socca into twelve 3-inch squares. You will need three slices for each serving.

Assemble the Socca:

1. Spoon a couple of tablespoons of marinara onto a plate and place a piece of socca on top.

2. Put 2 tablespoons of white bean puree on the socca slice and top with sautéed greens.

3. Place the next piece of socca on top of the bean puree and top with the greens.

4. Add the third slice of socca. Top with 1 tablespoon of bean puree, a tablespoon of marinara, and the caramelized leeks.

Hijiki Sea Cakes

Serves 4–6

These wholesome and delicious cakes are swimming with minerals from the sea. We top it with our version of a classic creamy tartar sauce that even people who never thought they liked tartar sauce will love.

1 lemon, for garnish

Preheat the oven to 350°F. Line a baking sheet with baking parchment.

Sea Cakes

1 (14-ounce) block firm
tofu, drained

¼ cup dry hijiki seaweed,
soaked in 4 cups water

½ medium-size onion,
finely diced

3 cloves garlic, sliced

1 tablespoon olive oil

Pinch of cayenne

1½ teaspoons dried dill

1 teaspoon dried thyme

1½ teaspoons Spike

1 tablespoon vegan
vegetable-flavor broth
powder, or ½ vegan
vegetable-flavor
bouillon cube

1½ teaspoons lemon juice

2 tablespoons mirin

1 tablespoon chopped
scallion

1 tablespoon chopped
fresh parsley, or
1 teaspoon dried

½ cup bread crumbs

Tartar Sauce

5 small dill pickles, cut into
small dice

1 tablespoon minced red
onion

1¼ teaspoons Spike

1½ teaspoons lemon zest

1 scallion, sliced

1 teaspoon chopped
fresh parsley, or
¼ teaspoon dried

¾ cup Vegenaise

1 small clove garlic

¾ teaspoon stone-ground
mustard

¾ teaspoon lemon juice

¼ teaspoon Florida Crystals

Make the Sea Cakes:

1. Crumble the tofu into a food processor. Pulse in the sea vegetables.

2. In a large skillet, sauté the onion and garlic in the oil until soft.

3. Add the herbs, spices, and broth powder to the pan and cook for 2 minutes. Transfer the mixture to the tofu mixture, pulsing until just combined.

4. In the sauté pan used for the onion mixture, combine the lemon juice and mirin, and raise the heat to medium-high. Stir the liquid for about a minute to deglaze the brown bits from the pan. Add this liquid to the ingredients in the food processor.

5. Process the tofu mixture in a food processor until smooth. Add the bread crumbs, chopped scallion, and parsley, and mix well.

6. Form the mixture into golf ball–size cakes, flatten slightly, and place on the prepared baking sheet. Bake for 15 minutes.

Make the Tartar Sauce:

1. While the cakes bake, mix all the sauce ingredients together in a bowl.

TO SERVE:
PLACE THE CAKES ON A PLATE DRESSED
WITH LEMON WEDGES AND A
SMALL SIDE OF THE TARTAR SAUCE.

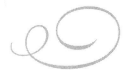

Herbed Tofu Loaf with Apple-Herb Stuffing and Cranberry-Orange Relish

Serves 4

This tofu loaf makes a great holiday entrée. We have served it to countless happy customers for many Thanksgivings, and now you can enjoy it at home. The moist, herbal stuffing gets its tart kick from the apple and its nutty crunch from the walnuts. It will remind you of the savory stuffings of Thanksgivings past, but without any of the poultry. And what Thanksgiving feast would be complete without cranberry relish? Here's our version.

Cranberry-Orange Relish

1½ cups fresh or frozen cranberries

1 cup maple syrup

1 cup orange juice

Zest of 1 medium-size orange

Zest and juice of 1 medium-size lemon

Pinch of sea salt

Apple-Herb Bread Stuffing

3 tablespoons extra-virgin olive oil

1 medium-size tart apple, peeled, cored, and diced

¼ cup walnuts

½ small white onion, minced

2 stalks celery, cut into ½-inch cubes

2 cloves garlic, minced

1 teaspoon dried thyme

1 teaspoon dried sage

1 teaspoon dried basil

4 cups stale bread, cubed

¼ cup stock

¼ teaspoon black pepper, or to taste

Sea salt

Make the Cranberry-Orange Relish:

1. In a medium-size saucepan over medium-high heat, combine the cranberries, maple syrup, and citrus juices and zests, and bring to a boil.

2. Lower the heat and cook until the cranberries pop, approximately 10 minutes. Add the salt and remove from the heat.

3. Chill and serve. If a thinner cranberry sauce is desired, blend in a blender or food processor until smooth.

Make the Apple-Herb Bread Stuffing:

1. In a medium-size saucepan, sauté the onion, apple, celery, and garlic in the oil. Add the herbs and walnuts and mix well.

2. Stir the bread into the mixture and pour in the stock. Mix all together well until moist. Add salt and pepper to taste.

Make the Herbed Tofu Loaf:

3 tablespoons extra-virgin olive oil, plus extra for oiling top of loaf

1 medium-size onion, cut into medium dice

2 cloves garlic, minced

2 (14-ounce) firm tofu blocks, drained and mashed

¾ cup nutritional yeast

3 tablespoons tamari

½ teaspoon black pepper

1 tablespoon dried thyme

1 tablespoon dried basil

2¼ cups Italian-style vegan bread crumbs

1 tablespoon white miso

Preheat the oven to 350°F. Oil a 9 by 3-inch loaf pan and line it with baking parchment. Set aside.

1. Heat the oil in a pan and sauté the onions and garlic until soft.

2. Combine the sautéed mixture and the remaining loaf ingredients in a food processor and mix well.

3. Divide the mixture in half and spread one-half in the bottom of the prepared pan, pressing down firmly with a spoon.

4. Spread ½ cup of the Apple-Herb Bread Stuffing evenly over the mixture in the loaf pan and top with the remaining tofu.

5. Oil the top of the loaf and bake for 25 to 30 minutes, or until firm to the touch.

6. Allow the loaf to cool 10 minutes, then turn out and serve sliced with Mushroom Gravy (page 58).

Love Bowl

Serves 1

Our signature Love Bowl is a hearty comfort food at its best. Enjoy!

1 cup cooked brown rice

½ cup cooked black beans

1 cup Sautéed Greens (page 65)

4 ounces Marinated Tempeh (page 55), or 4 slabs Baked Tofu, cut in half diagonally (page 53)

⅓ cup Peanut Sauce (page 59) or Mushroom Gravy (page 58)

Toasted sesame seeds, for garnish

Thinly sliced scallion, for garnish

1. Layer the rice, beans, greens, and tempeh in a medium-size serving bowl and top with your favorite sauce.

2. Serve hot, sprinkled with the sesame seeds and scallions.

Kevin's Tofu Murphy

Serves 4

1 (14-ounce) block
  extra-firm tofu, drained
2 tablespoons extra-virgin
  olive oil, for coating
3 medium-size Yukon Gold
  potatoes, quartered
¼ cup extra-virgin olive oil
1 large sweet onion, chopped
1 medium-size red bell
  pepper, chopped
1 medium-size green bell
  pepper, chopped
1 medium-size yellow bell
  pepper, chopped
10 cloves garlic, minced
2 medium-size portobello
  mushrooms, sliced
10 cherry peppers
2 teaspoons dried oregano
¼ teaspoon red pepper
  flakes (optional)
Salt and pepper
1 cup vegan vegetable
  stock (page 52)

Like a classic song that always gets you going, this dish will rock your taste buds. Kevin's version of the traditional Murphy will have you screaming encore!

Preheat the oven to 350°F.

1. Cut the tofu into bite-size cubes, coat lightly with olive oil, and bake for 10 to 15 minutes, until golden brown.

2. In a large sauté pan, sauté the potatoes in the ¼ cup of olive oil over medium heat for 10 minutes. Add the onion, bell peppers, garlic, and portobellos to the pan. Cook for 5 minutes.

3. Add the baked tofu, cherry peppers, oregano, red pepper flakes (if using), salt, pepper, and vegetable stock. Simmer for 10 minutes, or until the potatoes are fork tender.

Entrées

Pizza

Yield: Two 10-inch pizzas

With this convenient method for making pizza, you're on the road to pizza freedom. Try one of our suggestions or let your imagination be your guide.

1¼ cups warm water
1 teaspoon active dry yeast
1 teaspoon Sucanat
3 tablespoons extra-virgin olive oil
2 teaspoons sea salt
1 tablespoon Italian seasoning (see Spice Blends, page 23)
4 cups unbleached all-purpose flour

Suggested Toppings (or use any other vegetables you desire)

Vine-ripened tomatoes with fresh basil and olive oil

Sautéed spinach

Blanched broccoli

Roasted garlic (see step 1, page 123, for directions)

Artichoke hearts

Tofu Cheese (page 60)

House Marinara (page 58)

Tempeh Sausage (page 29)

Sautéed zucchini

1. In a medium-size bowl, combine the water, yeast, and Sucanat, and let the mixture rest in a warm spot for 5 minutes until it looks foamy.

2. Mix in the olive oil, salt, and seasoning. Add the flour slowly, stirring until the dough comes together. It should not be too sticky.

3. Turn out the dough onto a lightly floured work surface and knead for 10 minutes, until it is smooth and elastic.

4. Coat the inside of a bowl with 2 tablespoons of oil and place the dough inside, rolling it to coat all surfaces with oil. Cover the dough with plastic wrap and let rise for at least 1 or 2 hours in a warm, draft-free place until doubled.

5. Preheat the oven to 450°F.

6. Lightly knead the dough and divide in half. Cover one-half with a damp towel and shape the other half into a free-form circle.

7. Transfer the formed dough to a baking sheet or pizza stone, if you have one, and brush the crust with olive oil. Make sure to poke a few holes in the crust. Bake for 3 minutes.

8. Add the topping of your choice and bake for 10 minutes.

9. Prepare and bake the second pizza using the remaining dough.

Coconut Seitan

Serves 4–6

A taste of the islands—pan-fried Brazil nut–crusted coconut seitan, topped with a tart-sweet pineapple-mango chutney—this dish will make you feel the sun is shining even on the coldest day of the year.

1 pound seitan, sliced ½-inch thick

1½ cups canola or other flavorless oil, for frying

Pineapple-Mango Marmalade

1 cup chopped fresh pineapple

½ ripe mango, pitted, peeled, and diced

½ cup red onion, diced

1 tablespoon extra-virgin olive oil

½ teaspoon minced fresh sage, or ¼ teaspoon dried

1 medium-size roasted red pepper, chopped roughly

4 teaspoons agave nectar or rice syrup

1 tablespoon rice vinegar

1½ teaspoons fresh lemon juice

Pinch sea salt

Dredging Mixture

½ cup Brazil nuts

¼ cup unsweetened grated coconut

¾ cup unbleached all-purpose flour

½ teaspoon sea salt

Pinch of black pepper

Pinch of paprika

Wash

1 cup coconut milk or soy milk

2 tablespoons Vegenaise

Make the Pineapple-Mango Marmalade:

1. In a 2- to 3-quart saucepan, place all the marmalade ingredients and cook over medium heat until bubbling, stirring.

2. Turn down the heat and continue to stir, cooking for 15 to 20 minutes, or until the mixture has thickened slightly.

3. Remove from the heat and set aside to cool, to let the flavors marry.

Make the Dredging Mixture:

1. Grind the Brazil nuts in a food processor until crumbly.

2. Add the coconut, flour, salt, pepper, and paprika, and pulse for 1 more minute to incorporate.

3. Transfer the mixture to a shallow pan.

Make the Wash:

1. In another shallow pan, whisk together the coconut milk and Vegenaise.

Make the Seitan:

1. Dip the seitan slices in the wash, then coat each slice thoroughly in the dredging mixture to end up with a fairly dry piece of coated seitan.

2. In a large skillet, heat the oil over medium-high heat until hot. Test by tossing a crumb of dredging mixture into the oil—if it bubbles, the oil is ready.

3. Gently slip pieces of seitan into the oil and fry until golden. Transfer to paper towels to drain.

TO SERVE: SERVE WITH MASHED COCONUT YAMS (PAGE 62).

Entrées

Baked Samosas

Serves 4

A lighter version of the Indian classic, these samosas are baked and served as an entrée, crispy without the frying. They're filled with a wonderful melody of spiced potatoes, peas, and onions.

The tangy Banana-Ginger Chutney makes a wonderful accompaniment and can be made ahead of time; it keeps for about 3 weeks refrigerated.

Banana-Ginger Chutney
(recipe follows)

Tamarind Sauce
(recipe follows)

4 (9-inch) whole wheat tortillas

Samosa Filling

4 cups peeled and diced potatoes

2 tablespoons extra-virgin olive oil

1 small red onion, minced

3 cloves garlic, chopped

½ teaspoon ground coriander

1½ teaspoons mustard seeds

¾ teaspoon ground cumin

½ teaspoon curry powder

2 tablespoons Sucanat

¼ cup coconut milk

1 tablespoon lime juice

¼ teaspoon black pepper

¾ teaspoon sea salt

½ cup fresh or thawed frozen peas

Make the Samosa Filling:

1. Boil the potatoes until soft; then drain.

2. Heat the olive oil in a large saucepan, and cook the onion, garlic, and spices until the onions are soft. Add the Sucanat, coconut milk, and lime juice, and cook for 2 minutes more.

3. Mix in the potatoes and black pepper, and cook for 5 minutes more. Add the salt and the peas, and mix well.

Assemble the Samosas:

Preheat the oven to 425°F. Oil a baking sheet.

1. In the center of each tortilla, place approximately ½ cup of the samosa filling.

2. Fold the sides of each tortilla in toward the center and wrap the bottom up and over to form a rectangle. Cut across diagonally.

3. Place the samosa halves seam side down on the prepared baking sheet and brush the tops with a bit of oil.

4. Bake for 10 to 15 minutes, or until crispy. While the samosas bake, prepare the Tamarind Sauce.

5. Serve each samosa topped with some Banana-Ginger Chutney and Tamarind Sauce.

To create a substantial entrée, serve with seasonal vegetables atop Cashew Rice (page 56).

Banana-Ginger Chutney

1½ dried Anaheim chiles

3 medium-size bananas, chopped

½ medium-size onion, chopped into medium dice

½ medium-size apple, seeded and chopped into medium dice

¼ cup raisins

1 cup apple cider vinegar

¾ cup Sucanat

2 tablespoons minced fresh ginger

1½ tablespoons curry powder

Zest and juice of ½ medium-size lime

½ teaspoon sea salt

Tamarind Sauce

¼ cup tamarind pulp

2¼ teaspoons sea salt

1 teaspoon black pepper

2¼ cups Sucanat

¾ teaspoon cayenne

1½ tablespoons cumin seed, toasted and ground

2 cups water

Make the Banana-Ginger Chutney:

1. Rehydrate the chiles in hot water and rinse thoroughly to remove the seeds.

2. Combine the chiles and all the other ingredients in a 4- to 6-quart stockpot. Simmer over medium heat for 20 to 25 minutes, stirring often to prevent sticking. The chutney will start to darken and thicken.

3. Let cool and use as a condiment.

Will keep for 3 to 4 weeks, refrigerated in a tightly lidded container.

Make the Tamarind Sauce:

1. Place all the ingredients in a saucepan and bring to a boil.

2. Remove from the heat and set aside to cool.

Can be kept for several months refrigerated, and used to top rice, greens, and pretty much anything your heart desires.

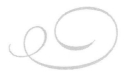

Seitan Satay

Serves 6

Cilantro Marinade
2 bunches fresh cilantro, washed well and chopped (leaves and stems)
1½ cups canola oil
1 cup rice syrup
¼ cup lemon juice
½ teaspoon salt
½ teaspoon black pepper

Satay
24 wooden or bamboo skewers, soaked in water for 15 minutes
6 cups seitan, cut in 1-inch pieces
½ cup Peanut Sauce (page 59)

This Thai-style marinated and grilled seitan served with a spicy peanut sauce dish is so delicious that even die-hard carnivores will come back for more!

Preheat a grill and lightly oil it.

Make the Cilantro Marinade:
1. Place all the ingredients in a blender and blend well.

Assemble the Satay:
1. Thread the seitan pieces onto the presoaked skewers, a few per skewer, and coat with the marinade.

2. Place the seitan sticks on the grill and cook, turning carefully once or twice, until the seitan is cooked through and lightly charred around the edges.

3. Remove the satay sticks from the grill and drizzle with the peanut sauce.

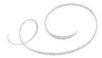

TO SERVE: ACCOMPANY WITH BROWN RICE AND SAUTÉED SEASONAL VEGETABLES.

Southern-Style Seitan

Serves 6

Maple-Mustard Sauce
½ cup stone-ground mustard
3 tablespoons extra-virgin olive oil
4½ teaspoons tamari
½ cup maple syrup
4½ teaspoons water

You don't have to live in the South to create fabulous Southern-style cuisine. It's the seven herbs and spices brought together in Cajun spice that really make the flavor of this dish—crisp seitan nuggets served with a tangy Maple-Mustard Sauce and sautéed greens.

Make the Maple-Mustard Sauce:
1. Put all the sauce ingredients into a blender, blend until smooth, and set aside.

Seitan

6 cups seitan, torn into nuggets

1½ cups plus 2 tablespoons unbleached all-purpose flour

¼ cup Cajun spice (see Spice Blends, page 24)

¾ teaspoon total, mixed salt and pepper

1½ cups canola oil, for frying

Make the Seitan:

1. In a large bowl, coat the seitan nuggets with flour. Add the Cajun spice mixture to the bowl and recoat the seitan. Season with salt and pepper.

2. Heat the oil in a large skillet and fry the seitan nuggets in small batches until crisp. Transfer the cooked nuggets to paper towels to drain.

3. Sprinkle with more Cajun spice and salt and pepper to taste.

TO SERVE:
SERVE WITH MAPLE-MUSTARD SAUCE,
SAUTÉED GREENS (PAGE 65),
AND ROASTED YAMS (PAGE 64).

Thai Coconut Tempeh Stix

Serves 4–6

This dish is inspired by the flavors of Thailand.

Basil-Lemongrass Sauce

¼ cup sliced fresh ginger

4 cloves garlic

2 tablespoons chopped fresh basil

4 pieces star anise

3 tablespoons chopped fresh lemongrass

1 (15-ounce) can coconut milk

1½ cups water

1½ tablespoons vegan vegetable-flavor broth powder

1½ teaspoons sea salt

3 tablespoons kudzu

⅔ cup water

2 tablespoons rice syrup

Make the Basil-Lemongrass Sauce:

1. Place the ginger, garlic, basil, star anise, and lemongrass in a piece of washed cheesecloth and tie securely.

2. Place the cheesecloth bundle, coconut milk, water, salt, and broth powder in a saucepan, bring to a simmer, and cook for 20 minutes.

3. Remove the cheesecloth bundle from the pan and press the liquid back into the saucepan through a strainer.

4. Make a kudzu slurry by mixing the kudzu and the water in a small container.

5. Add the slurry and the rice syrup to the saucepan and simmer for an additional 10 minutes. Remove from the heat and set aside.

Thai Bread Crumbs
1¼ cups dried bread
   crumbs

1 cup sesame seeds

¼ cup unsweetened
   coconut flakes

Tempeh Stix
8 ounces Marinated
   Tempeh (page 55)

TO SERVE:
SERVE WITH THE
REMAINING
BASIL-LEMONGRASS
SAUCE AND
CASHEW RICE
(PAGE 56).

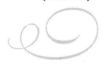

3 medium-size yams,
   peeled and cut into
   bite-size chunks

2 tablespoons extra-virgin
   olive oil

1 teaspoon garlic powder

2 pounds lasagna noodles

6 cups House Marinara
   (page 58)

8 ounces baby spinach,
   washed well

3 cups Tofu Cheese
   (page 60)

Make the Thai Bread Crumbs:

1. In a medium-size bowl, combine the bread crumbs, sesame seeds, and coconut flakes.

Make the Tempeh Stix:

Preheat the oven to 375°F. Oil a baking sheet and set aside.

1. Cut the marinated tempeh in half and cut each half into three sticks.

2. In one medium-size bowl, place ½ cup of the Basil-Lemongrass Sauce; in another, place the Thai Bread Crumbs.

3. Submerge the tempeh sticks in the bowl of sauce, shake off any excess, and roll each of the stix in the crumbs until completely coated.

4. Place the stix on the prepared baking sheet and bake for 15 minutes, or until golden.

Vegetable Lasagne

Serves 6

From grandparents to kids, who doesn't love this family favorite? It's easy to prepare in any season using whatever fresh vegetables the market has to offer. In summer, grill the vegetables for an extra layer of flavor, or try roasted vegetables, such as zucchini and summer squash. This is a good recipe to make ahead. It can also be frozen and is great for a buffet.

Preheat the oven to 350°F. Oil a 9 by 13-inch baking dish and set aside. Line a baking sheet with baking parchment.

1. Place the yams in a medium-size bowl and toss with the oil and garlic powder.

2. Spread the yams on the prepared baking sheet and bake for 15 to 20 minutes, until soft and golden. Sprinkle with salt and pepper while still hot.

3. While the yams bake, cook the lasagna noodles according to package directions and drain.

4. Spread 1 cup of House Marinara over the bottom of the baking dish and cover with a layer of five overlapping lasagna noodles. Scatter one-third of the spinach and one-third of the roasted yams over the noodles, then top with one-quarter of the tofu cheese.

5. Repeat twice more, layering the noodles, spinach, yams, and cheese in that order. Pour 1 cup of marinara over all, then place the last layer of noodles on top.

6. Mix 1 cup of marinara with the fourth quarter of the tofu cheese and spread over the top of the lasagne.

7. Cover with foil and bake for 15 minutes; then remove the foil and bake for an additional 15 minutes.

8. Remove from the oven and let rest for 10 minutes before cutting and serving.

To prepare ahead, simply bake and chill. This reheats well and will keep for 4 days in the refrigerator, or 3 to 4 weeks in the freezer. To reheat, thaw, if frozen, cover with foil, and bake in a preheated oven at 400°F for 15 minutes covered, remove the foil, and bake for another 10 minutes.

Potato, Green Onion, and Rosemary Spelt Gnocchi

Serves 4-6

3 medium-size russet
  potatoes

1½ teaspoons sea salt, plus
  extra for cooking pasta

3 cups whole-grain spelt
  flour, plus extra for
  mixing and rolling

¼ cup extra-virgin olive oil

2 scallions, minced

¼ teaspoon black pepper

1 teaspoon fresh rosemary

These little dumplings, made of simple ingredients, are comforting and filling. They can be topped with any of your favorite sauces, including pesto, our House Marinara (page 58), or even just olive oil, garlic, and parsley. This version is made with whole-grain spelt flour, which can be easier on those who have wheat sensitivities.

Preheat the oven to 400°F.

1. Wrap the potatoes in foil and bake for about 1 hour, or until tender. Peel the potatoes when completely cool.

2. In a large bowl, mash the cooled potatoes and the 1½ teaspoons of salt. Add about a cup of the spelt flour and mix together. Add 3 tablespoons of the olive oil; the scallions, pepper, and rosemary; and the remaining spelt flour. Mix the dough together until it is no longer sticky, adding more spelt flour if needed.

3. Heat a large pot of liberally salted water to a boil. Set near the pot a plate oiled with the remaining tablespoon of olive oil.

4. Divide the dough into six equal pieces. On a floured surface, roll out each piece into a long snake about 1 inch in diameter.

5. Cut each rope into twenty to twenty-five ½-inch gnocchi and let rest for a moment.

6. Add about fifteen gnocchi to the boiling water, in batches. Cook for at least 5 minutes, removing each piece with a slotted spoon once it floats to the top of the pot, making sure to drain off as much water as possible. Set the drained gnocchi on the oiled plate.

7. When the gnocchi cool a little, they firm up and can be pan-fried for an extra touch. They can also be made ahead, refrigerated, and eaten the next day.

White Bean Crepes with Balsamic Grilled Tempeh and Basil "Butter"

Serves 6

In this recipe we've used white beans for the filling, but have fun with this versatile crepe recipe. Fill it with your favorite vegetables or fruit compotes.

Balsamic Grilled Tempeh
(recipe follows)

Basil "Butter" (recipe
follows)

Crepes

1 cup unbleached
all-purpose flour

3 tablespoons gluten flour

2 teaspoons Sucanat

½ teaspoon sea salt

2 tablespoons canola oil

2 cups water

Filling

2 tablespoons extra-virgin
olive oil

5 cloves garlic

3 cups baby spinach,
washed

2 cups cooked white beans,
or 1 (15-ounce) can,
drained and rinsed

½ teaspoon sea salt

Pinch of black pepper

CHEF'S TIP:
PREPARE THE BALSAMIC
GRILLED TEMPEH BEFORE
STARTING THE CREPES.

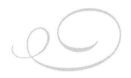

Preheat the oven to 250°F.

Make the Crepes:

1. In a medium-size bowl, whisk together the dry ingredients. Add the oil and water, and whisk to combine. The batter should be thin.

2. Heat a small amount of oil in a 7-inch nonstick sauté pan over medium heat.

3. Pour ¼ cup of batter into the center of the pan and swirl to coat the bottom of the pan. When bubbles appear on top and the edges are brown, flip the crepe and lightly brown the other side. Transfer to a foil-covered plate and repeat with the remaining crepes.

4. Keep the cooked crepes warm, covered, in a 250°F oven until ready to use.

Make the Filling:

1. Sauté the garlic in olive oil over low heat. When browned, remove from the pan and set aside.

2. Sauté the spinach in the same oil until wilted, remove from the heat, and let cool.

3. Chop together the garlic and spinach, mix into the white beans, and add the salt and pepper.

Balsamic Grilled Tempeh

1 teaspoon hot sauce

2 tablespoons extra-virgin olive oil

2 tablespoons balsamic vinegar

1 teaspoon dried rosemary

1 teaspoon Italian seasoning (see Spice Blends, page 23)

1 tablespoon stone-ground mustard

1 pound tempeh, cut in four equal pieces

Basil "Butter"

1 bunch fresh basil

¼ cup vegan margarine

1 tablespoon extra-virgin olive oil

½ teaspoon pepper

Assemble the Crepes:

1. In the center of each crepe, place a generous ¼-cup scoop of the bean filling.

2. Roll each crepe and place three on each plate, then put two pieces of grilled tempeh on top of them. Drizzle with Basil "Butter" and serve hot.

Make the Balsamic Grilled Tempeh:

1. Process the hot sauce, oil, vinegar, rosemary, Italian seasoning, and mustard in a blender until smooth.

2. Pour the mixture over the tempeh pieces and let them marinate for 1 hour or more.

3. Oil and preheat a grill. Grill the tempeh on both sides and return it to the marinade. If no grill is available, place the tempeh under a broiler and broil until slightly charred, flipping once to ensure even browning.

4. When ready to use, cut the tempeh into twelve equal pieces.

Make the Basil "Butter":

1. Blanch the basil briefly in salted boiling water, and shock in ice water to brighten the color. Drain well.

2. Process the basil, margarine, oil, and pepper in a blender and chill. Serve cold on the hot crepes.

TO SERVE:
SERVE WITH ROASTED TOMATO,
BASIL, AND CORN SALAD
(PAGE 92).

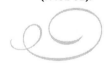

Wild Rice
Risotto Cakes

Serves 4

1 large yellow onion, or
3 shallots, cut into
small dice

2 carrots, peeled and cut
into small dice

3 stalks celery, cut into
small dice

3 cloves garlic, minced

1 tablespoon dried thyme

1 tablespoon dried basil

1 cup long-grain brown rice

½ cup wild rice

7 cups vegan vegetable stock
(page 52), warmed

½ cup white wine

2 tablespoons finely
chopped fresh parsley

1 tablespoon vegan
margarine

¾ cup bread crumbs

Leek and Red Pepper
Sauce (recipe follows)

The wild rice adds a pleasing crunch to these risotto cakes, and the brown rice makes them exceptionally nutritious. Serve these cakes with some grilled tempeh and sautéed greens for a savory and satisfying meal, or make mini cakes for an elegant appetizer.

Preheat the oven to 350°F. Line a baking sheet with baking parchment and oil the paper.

1. In a heavy saucepan over medium-low heat, sauté the onion, carrots, celery, and garlic with 2 tablespoons of the olive oil for approximately 8 minutes, until softened. Add the dried herbs and both rices, and stir to coat.

2. Add 1 cup of warm stock and stir over medium heat until all the liquid is absorbed. Repeat, stirring constantly, until all the stock is absorbed.

3. After the last cup of stock is absorbed, add the ½ cup of white wine and stir until that is absorbed. Stir in the fresh parsley, and then the vegan margarine. Add ¼ cup of the bread crumbs, and mix well.

4. Spread out the risotto on a plate or baking sheet and let sit until cooled.

5. Wet your hands, scoop out ½ cup of the mixture at a time, and form into balls. Space the balls well apart on the prepared baking sheet and lightly sprinkle with one-half of the remaining bread crumbs. Lightly flatten the risotto into ½-inch-thick cakes, then sprinkle the tops with the last of the bread crumbs.

6. Bake for 15 to 20 minutes, or until golden. Drain on paper towels. While they cook, prepare the Leek and Red Pepper Sauce.

7. Serve with the Leek and Red Pepper Sauce.

Leek and Red Pepper Sauce

2 medium-size white
onions, cut into
small dice

1 tablespoon minced garlic

2 leeks, split in half,
washed well and
sliced thinly

2 tablespoons plus
1 teaspoon vegan
margarine

6 roasted red peppers,
sliced thinly

2 tablespoons vegan
vegetable-flavor broth
powder or 1 vegan
vegetable-flavor bouil-
lon cube, dissolved in
½ cup water

½ teaspoon dried dill

2 teaspoons minced
scallion

Pinch of sea salt

Pinch of black pepper

Minced fresh parsley,
for garnish

Make the Leek and Red Pepper Sauce:

1. In a small saucepan over medium heat, sauté the onions, garlic, and leeks in 2 tablespoons of the margarine until soft.

2. Add the red peppers, broth, and dill, and sauté for about 2 minutes. Remove from the heat.

3. With an immersion blender, pulse until the ingredients combine to create a bright sauce. Stir in the remaining teaspoon of margarine and sprinkle liberally with minced parsley.

Live Foods

There are many different definitions of raw or "live" foods. Our definition of a raw food diet is one that is free of animal products and includes fruits, vegetables, nuts, and seeds—none of which are heated above 108°F. Proponents of raw foods believe that when we eat cooked food, our body uses up its own enzymes that it has worked hard to produce and store. Enzymes help us to digest and assimilate everything we eat, giving us energy and health benefits. Cooking foods destroys the enzymes that they contain. By adding to our diet raw foods whose enzymes are intact, we aid in the digestive process and give our body a much-needed break, saving those valuable digestive enzymes for that extra-big piece of vegan Chocolate Ganache cake when we splurge!

Nuts and seeds pack raw foods with protein and good fats, too. Avocado, a rich source of healthy vegan fat, can be a key ingredient in countless sauces, raw soups, salads, dips, or even a raw fruit smoothie. We use dehydrators for some of these recipes, such as the Pizza Crackers, but try any of the cheeses or sauces with cabbage leaves or crisp romaine.

A perfect example of using live vegetables instead of cooked is the Leaf Wrap filled with guacamole and zesty sun-dried tomato pâté.

This section offers recipes for both savory and sweet dishes, from the Raw Herb Vegetable Croquette to the Raw Apple Pie with Raw Cream Whipped Topping. You don't have to adopt an all–raw food diet to reap the benefits; however, these recipes are so packed with good taste, your oven might stay off for a while after you try them.

Adam's Pink Lady Apple Salsa

Serves 6

3 medium-size Pink Lady apples, cored and cut into small dice

¼ cup minced fresh cilantro

¼ cup minced fresh mint

½ cup thinly sliced scallions

1 medium-size jalapeño, seeded and minced

Zest and juice of 2 limes

Pinch of sea salt

"Pink Lady apples are my favorite because of their balanced flavor. They are usually quite tart, a bit sweet, crisp, and beautifully colored. This salsa is delicious on spinach salads or as a refreshing complement to a grilled tofu or seitan dish."

—*Adam*

1. Toss the ingredients together and refrigerate for at least 1 hour in a covered container.

2. Toss again prior to use, to coat with juices and marry the flavors.

Curried Almond Pâté

Yield: 1 cup; serves 4

½ cup raw almonds, soaked overnight

1 clove garlic

1½ teaspoons chopped scallion

¼ cup extra-virgin olive oil

½ teaspoon curry powder

1 teaspoon nama shoyu

2 tablespoons water

1½ teaspoons chopped fresh cilantro

¾ teaspoon light agave syrup

Almonds are the perfect, easily digestible nut for humans, especially after soaking. This pâté will fill you up and is chock-full of protein, calcium, and great flavor. Serve it in napa cabbage leaves with the Fennel-Apple Dressing (page 80).

1. In a food processor, process the garlic, scallions, curry powder, and water until evenly incorporated. With the motor running, slowly add the soaked almonds through the chute. Stop the machine halfway through to scrape down the sides.

2. Add the olive oil and nama shoyu, and pulse until incorporated. Add the cilantro and agave syrup, and blend until smooth.

3. Transfer the mixture to a covered container and refrigerate for a couple of hours to allow the flavors to marry.

Flaxseed Crackers

Yield: Twelve 2-inch-square crackers

Sesame seeds bring calcium to this savory, crisp dehydrated cracker, and fiber and omegas are delivered by the flaxseeds. Try using the same base recipe to experiment with a variety of seasonings.

1 cup raw sesame seeds
1 cup flaxseeds
2 cups water
1½ teaspoons garlic powder
1½ teaspoons sea salt
1½ teaspoons minced fresh ginger
2 tablespoons minced scallion
¼ cup nutritional yeast

1. Combine all the ingredients and soak for at least 15 minutes, until the mixture thickens and becomes gel-like.

2. Halve the mixture and spread thinly onto two Teflex dehydrator sheets.

3. Score the dough into twelve crackers and dehydrate at 115°F for at least 12 hours. The crackers should be crisp when done.

Leaf Wraps

Serves 6–8

This combination of Brazil nuts and sun-dried tomatoes layered with avocados, fresh tomatoes, and shredded spinach is as delectable as it is colorful. We use the nutritious and versatile Sprinkle "Cheese" on top to add a zest that makes these reminiscent of tacos.

1 head romaine lettuce, washed and separated into leaves
½ cup fresh tomatoes, diced
½ cup spinach, shredded
1 avocado, sliced into thin pieces
Sun-Dried Tomato Pâté (recipe follows)
Sprinkle "Cheese" (page 60)

1. Spoon 2 tablespoons of Sun-Dried Tomato Pâté into the center of each leaf. On top of the pâté, layer 2 avocado slices, 1 tablespoon spinach, and 1 tablespoon tomatoes.

2. Serve four to a plate and sprinkle liberally with Sprinkle "Cheese."

Sun-Dried Tomato Pâté

Yield: 1 pint

¼ cup sun-dried tomatoes

6 tablespoons raw
sunflower seeds

½ cup Brazil nuts

1½ cloves garlic

1 tablespoon chopped
fresh parsley

2 tablespoons chopped
scallions

2 tablespoons extra-virgin
olive oil

Zest and juice from
¼ large lemon

¼ teaspoon freshly ground
black pepper

Pinch of cayenne

2 tablespoons chopped
black olives

1. Soak the sun-dried tomatoes in 1 cup of warm water until soft, about 1 hour. Drain, reserving the soaking liquid.

2. In a food processor, blend the sunflower seeds and Brazil nuts until finely ground. Transfer to a bowl and set aside.

3. Combine in the food processor ¾ cup of the reserved soaking water, the sun-dried tomatoes, and the rest of the ingredients except for 1 tablespoon of black olives and the reserved nuts, and process until smooth.

4. Add the processed nuts and blend until smooth. Stir in the remaining black olives.

Will keep for 4 to 5 days refrigerated.

Live Lasagne

Serves 6

Zucchini Noodles

2 medium-size summer
squash

3 medium-size zucchini

¼ cup fresh lemon juice

1 tablespoon extra-virgin
olive oil

½ teaspoon sea salt

To Assemble:

Raw Cashew Cheese
(recipe follows)

2 cups baby spinach,
washed

1 large portobello mushroom cap, thinly sliced

Live Tomato Sauce (recipe
follows)

½ cup Sprinkle "Cheese"
(page 60)

A show-stopping live entrée, this creamy light lasagne uses cashews to create a cheeselike spread layered with fresh yellow squash, zucchini, and sweet sun-dried tomato sauce. Prepare the lasagne in a large glass baking dish and cut into serving portions, or stack into a free-form individual sculptural masterpiece for each guest.

Make the Zucchini Noodles:

1. Cut the ends off the squash, and then cut them in half width-wise. Slice as thinly as possible lengthwise using a knife or mandoline.

2. In a bowl, mix together the lemon juice, olive oil, and salt.

3. Place the squash strips in the lemon marinade and set aside for 10 to 15 minutes.

153

To Assemble the Lasagne:

1. Drain the squash and blot dry with a clean towel.

2. Lightly oil an 8-inch square baking dish. Arrange the squash noodles neatly along the bottom of the dish. Spread half of the cashew cheese evenly over the noodles.

3. Arrange the spinach leaves and mushroom slices evenly on top of the cashew cheese and press into the cheese. Spoon one-third of the tomato sauce over the spinach and mushrooms.

4. Arrange another layer of squash noodles over the top and repeat the cheese, mushroom, spinach, and tomato sauce layers.

5. Arrange the final layer of noodles, top with tomato sauce, and sprinkle with Sprinkle "Cheese."

Raw Cashew Cheese

Yield: 1 cup

1 cup raw cashews

2 cups water

1 clove garlic, chopped

¼ cup nutritional yeast

1 teaspoon fresh lemon juice

¼ teaspoon sea salt

Pinch freshly ground black pepper

¼ teaspoon nama shoyu

1. Soak the raw cashews for 20 minutes in 1½ cups of the water. Drain and rinse.

2. In a food processor, blend the cashews and the remaining ½ cup of water until creamy.

3. Add the garlic and yeast and blend well, pausing to scrape down the sides of the processor container. Add the remaining ingredients and mix well, pausing to scrape down the sides.

Will keep for 4 days refrigerated.

Live Tomato Sauce

Yield: 2 cups

1 cup sun-dried tomatoes

¾ cup warm water

1 small tomato, seeded and chopped

½ teaspoon Italian seasoning (see Spice Blends, page 23)

¼ cup nutritional yeast

¼ cup extra-virgin olive oil

¾ teaspoon sea salt

2 teaspoons fresh lemon juice

1. Soak the sun-dried tomatoes in the warm water for 20 minutes.

2. In a food processor or blender, blend the water and sun-dried tomatoes until smooth.

3. Add the remaining ingredients and blend well, pausing occasionally to scrape down the sides of the machine until the mixture is smooth.

Will keep for 4 days refrigerated.

Live Nachos

Serves 6–8

1 cup Live Salsa (page 156)

Nacho Chips

1½ cups raw sunflower seeds

2 cups ground flaxseeds

½ cup ground sesame seeds

1 tablespoon taco seasoning mix (see Spice Blends, page 23)

1 tablespoon ground cumin

½ teaspoon sea salt

2 tablespoons nama shoyu

¼ cup minced fresh cilantro

½ cup fresh lime juice

½ cup nutritional yeast

3 scallions, sliced thinly

2 teaspoons minced fresh oregano

1 large jalapeño, seeded and minced

These zesty nachos are great as a starter or as a whole entrée. You won't believe that this simple blend of ingredients can make something so outrageous. A blend of cashews, parsley, and nutritional yeast creates the smooth texture of the topper.

Make the Chips:

1. Soak the sunflower seeds for 2 hours in enough water to cover.

2. Drain and rinse the sunflower seeds, then purée in a food processor.

3. Add the flaxseeds and sesame seeds to the food processor with all the remaining chip ingredients. Process until the mixture becomes a slurry, adding a little water as needed to make it a spreadable consistency.

4. Spread thinly onto Teflex dehydrator sheets, score into chips roughly 2 by 3 inches, and dehydrate for 8 hours at 115°F. Gently peel off the chips, flip them over, and return them to the dehydrator until crunchy, about 4 more hours.

Raw Sour Cream

¼ cup raw cashews

2 cups plus 2 tablespoons water

¼ cup fresh lemon juice

2 tablespoons apple cider vinegar

½ teaspoon sea salt

¼ cup chopped fresh parsley

Make the Raw Sour Cream:

1. Soak the cashews in 2 cups of the water for 1 hour. Drain and rinse well.

2. Blend the cashews and all the remaining ingredients in a blender or food processor to a smooth cream.

Assemble the Nachos:

1. Place the chips on a plate, cover with salsa, and top with sour cream.

Extra chips can be stored in an airtight container for about 3 weeks or can be frozen for up to 2 months.

Live Salsa

Yield: 5 cups

A delicious, fat-free accompaniment to our nachos, live nachos, and potato skins. A fresh jalapeño will add fire.

4 medium-size ripe tomatoes, diced

10 cloves garlic, minced

1 small red onion, minced

1 small white onion, minced

3 scallions, minced

¼ cup finely chopped fresh cilantro

¼ cup fresh lime juice

¼ cup apple cider vinegar

1 teaspoon agave syrup

¾ teaspoon sea salt

½ teaspoon black pepper

Pinch of cayenne

½ medium-size jalapeño, minced (optional)

Variations

Add 1 cup diced fresh pineapple

or 1 cup fresh corn

or 1 cup diced jicama

1. Mix all the ingredients together and allow the flavors to marry.

Live Pizza Crackers

Serves 4

These lively, fun crackers, made of pumpkin seeds, buckwheat, sunflower seeds, sun-dried tomatoes, carrots, Italian herbs, and spices, can be a filling meal in themselves or a great starter. You can top these with cashew cheese, sun-dried tomato sauce, dark greens marinated in olive oil, and spiral-cut yams or zucchini, and finish with a tiny bit of sun-dried black olives and the indispensable Sprinkle "Cheese."

Raw Pizza Crackers
1 cup ground flaxseeds
1 cup buckwheat groats
1 cup raw pumpkin seeds
1 cup raw sunflower seeds
1 cup chopped carrots
2 cups chopped sun-dried tomatoes
½ cup raw sesame seeds
1½ teaspoons dried thyme
1½ teaspoons dried basil
1½ teaspoons garlic powder
1½ teaspoons onion powder
3 cups water
1 teaspoon sea salt

Marinated Greens
2 tablespoons apple cider vinegar
1 tablespoon extra-virgin olive oil
¼ teaspoon sea salt
3 leaves kale or dark green of choice, washed and chopped finely
2 tablespoons Sprinkle "Cheese" (page 60)
2 cups Live Tomato Sauce (page 155)
1 cup Raw Cashew Cheese (page 154)
½ cup grated or spiralized zucchini
6 sun-dried black olives, chopped

Make the Crackers:
1. Combine all the cracker ingredients, cover with the water, and allow the liquid to absorb.

2. Run the mixture through any masticating juicer or process in a food processor until mostly smooth with some texture.

3. Spread the mixture thinly onto a Teflex dehydrator sheet and score the crackers into 2-inch squares. Place in the dehydrator at 115°F for 8 hours. Flip over and continue to dehydrate for an additional 4 to 6 hours, until the crackers are crunchy.

Assemble the Pizza Crackers:
1. Whisk together the vinegar, oil, and salt. Pour over the greens and let marinate for 10 or more minutes.

2. Lay out the crackers and top each with 1 teaspoon of Live Tomato Sauce and 2 teaspoons of Raw Cashew Cheese.

3. Top each cracker with a generous sprinkling of kale, some grated zucchini, and 1 teaspoon of black olives. Finish with Sprinkle "Cheese."

These crackers can be stored in an airtight container for several weeks and are an appetizing addition to any salad.

CHEF'S TIP: THESE MINI PIZZAS
SHOULD NOT BE ASSEMBLED
TOO FAR IN ADVANCE OR THEY
WILL BECOME SOGGY.

Raw Cheese Trio

Serves 4–6

This is a trio like no other: Smoky Cashew-Pecan-Garlic Cheese, Cashew–Brazil Nut–Pumpkin Seed Herb Cheese, and Cashew–Brazil Nut–Tomato–Fennel Cheese. Serve these on a bed of baby field greens with golden Flax Crackers, fresh apple slices, and grapes for a mouth-watering culinary creation.

Flaxseed Crackers (page 152)

To Prepare the Smoky Cashew-Pecan-Garlic Cheese:

1. Drain and rinse both kinds of nuts. Transfer to a food processor and process until the mixture forms a paste. Add the curry, umeboshi paste, garlic, water, oil, and agave, and blend until smooth. Add the salt and dulse and blend to incorporate.

2. Chill the mixture. Form into Ping-Pong-size balls, then flatten and form into wheels. Coat them with the chopped nut mixture.

To Prepare the Cashew–Brazil Nut– Pumpkin Seed Herb Cheese:

1. Drain and rinse the seeds and nuts. Transfer to a food processor and process until the mixture forms a paste. Add the oil, water, herbs, garlic, and umeboshi paste, and blend until smooth.

2. Chill the mixture. Form into wheels, as above.

Smoky Cashew-Pecan-Garlic Cheese

1 cup raw pecans, soaked overnight

⅔ cup raw cashews, soaked overnight

½ teaspoon curry powder

1 teaspoon umeboshi plum paste

2 cloves garlic, minced

1 tablespoon water

1 tablespoon extra-virgin olive oil

½ teaspoon agave

⅛ teaspoon sea salt

⅛ teaspoon dulse flakes

¼ cup raw pecans, chopped, for garnish

Cashew–Brazil Nut–Pumpkin Seed Herb Cheese

3 cups raw pumpkin seeds, soaked overnight

1 cup Brazil nuts, soaked overnight

½ cup raw cashews, soaked overnight

¼ cup extra-virgin olive oil

¼ cup water

1 tablespoon chopped fresh savory

1 tablespoon chopped fresh sage

2 tablespoons chopped fresh parsley

½ cup chopped fresh dill

2 cloves garlic

2 tablespoons umeboshi plum paste

Cashew–Brazil Nut–Tomato–Fennel Cheese

3 cups raw cashews, soaked overnight

1½ cups Brazil nuts, soaked overnight

½ cup extra-virgin olive oil

1 cup sun-dried tomatoes, soaked overnight, reserve soaking water

¼ cup nutritional yeast

¼ medium-size yellow onion

½ teaspoon fennel seeds

1 tablespoon umeboshi plum paste

2 tablespoons agave

2 tablespoons chopped scallion

To Prepare the Cashew–Brazil Nut–Tomato–Fennel Cheese:

1. Drain and rinse both kinds of nuts. Transfer to a food processor and process until the mixture forms a paste. Add the oil, sun-dried tomatoes, yeast, onion, fennel seeds, umeboshi paste, and agave, and blend, gradually adding the reserved soaking water until smooth.

2. Chill, form into small wheels, and coat them with the chopped scallions, as described above.

Live Foods

Raw Herb-Vegetable Croquette

Yield: 28 croquettes; serves 7

A blend of walnuts, sunflower seeds, pumpkin seeds, carrots, cilantro, and spices slowly dehydrated to create a crisp patty, this croquette is packed with calcium, zinc, and beta-carotene, plus savory herbs that help cleanse and detoxify the blood. Top the croquette with creamy Raw Cashew Aioli and serve it over a bed of greens for a refreshing, satisfying meal. You can also serve this on Pizza Crackers (page 157) with lettuce and fresh tomato for an on-the-go sandwich.

1 cup raw walnuts

1 cup raw sunflower seeds

1 cup raw pumpkin seeds

1 cup roughly chopped small pieces of broccoli

1 cup shredded carrots

½ cup diced red onion, rinsed

2 cloves garlic, chopped

¼ cup chopped fresh parsley

¼ cup chopped fresh cilantro

1 tablespoon chopped fresh oregano

2 tablespoons fennel seeds

1 teaspoon black pepper

1 lemon, juiced

3 tablespoons extra-virgin olive oil

2 teaspoons sea salt

2 teaspoons miso

Spring greens, for serving

Raw Cashew Aioli (recipe follows)

1. Soak the walnuts and sunflower and pumpkin seeds together in 5 cups of water for 2 hours. Drain and rinse well.

2. In a food processor, finely chop the broccoli, carrots, onion, garlic, parsley, and cilantro. Add the fennel seeds, oregano, and black pepper, then add the olive oil, salt, lemon juice, and soaked seeds. Process, scraping down the sides with a rubber spatula as needed to create a smooth mixture.

3. To form croquettes, measure out ¼ cup of the mixture, place on a nonstick dehydrator sheet, and press down gently. Dehydrate at 115°F for 12 to 16 hours, flipping the croquettes over halfway through the process.

4. Serve on a bed of spring greens, three per plate, drizzled with Raw Cashew Aioli.

CHEF'S TIP: THESE CROQUETTES WILL KEEP WELL, REFRIGERATED, FOR UP TO A WEEK AND CAN BE FROZEN IN AN AIRTIGHT CONTAINER FOR 2 MONTHS.

Raw Cashew Aioli

Yield: 1½ cups

This creamy sauce is rich and velvety smooth and goes well with the croquettes. Thin it out a bit with water to use as a raw Alfredo sauce over spaghetti-sliced zucchini or as a delicious dip for any vegetables.

1 cup raw cashews, soaked overnight
½ cup water
1 clove garlic
¼ teaspoon sea salt
⅛ teaspoon dried marjoram
3 tablespoons extra-virgin olive oil
1½ teaspoons chopped scallion
½ teaspoon umeboshi plum paste
½ teaspoon nutritional yeast

1. Drain and rinse the soaked cashews.
2. Process all the ingredients together in a blender until smooth.

TO SERVE: YOU CAN CREATE A RAW NOODLE ENTRÉE BY SPIRALIZING A ZUCCHINI OR SUMMER SQUASH, TOSSING IN THIS AIOLI, AND TOPPING WITH SPRINKLE "CHEESE" FOR A NICE FINISH.

Raw Maki Hand Roll

Serves 8

Crisp nori are filled with creamy Brazil Nut Pâté layered with spinach, thin strips of carrots, zucchini, and shredded cabbage.
Feel free to use any seasonal fresh vegetables and roll.
Serve with zesty Miso-Wasabi Dip.

Brazil Nut Pâté
Yield: 1½ cups
¾ cup raw pumpkin seeds, soaked overnight
¾ cup Brazil nuts, soaked overnight
1 clove garlic
2 tablespoons flaxseed oil
½ cup water
Pinch of cayenne
Zest and juice of ½ medium-size lemon
¼ teaspoon sea salt

Make the Brazil Nut Pâté:

1. Drain and rinse the pumpkin seeds and Brazil nuts. Process them with the garlic in a food processor until finely ground. Add the oil and water to the processor and blend until the mixture is smooth.

2. Add the cayenne, lemon juice and zest, and salt, and blend for at least 2 to 3 minutes until smooth.

Miso–Wasabi Dip
Yield: 2 cups

¼ cup miso

1½ cups warm water

1 teaspoon ground ginger

½ cup wasabi powder

2 tablespoons mirin

1 tablespoon black
   sesame seeds

To Assemble

4 sheets nori

1 medium-size carrot,
   cut into matchsticks

1 medium-size avocado,
   sliced

8 sweet pea shoots

10 spinach leaves,
   chopped

Make the Miso-Wasabi Dip:

1. Process all the dip ingredients except the sesame seeds in a blender.

2. Stir in the sesame seeds.

Assemble the Maki Hand Rolls:

1. Cut the nori sheets in half. Lay the sheet lengthwise in front of you.

2. Smear 1 tablespoon of the pâté on an angle from the bottom center of the nori sheet to the top left-hand corner. Lay the cut vegetables along the smear.

3. Fold the bottom left corner over the ingredients toward the top center and tuck under the ingredients. Roll the sheet toward the center right edge. Moisten the bottom right-hand corner to seal. Repeat with the remaining ingredients.

Live Buckwheat-Hempseed Granola Crunch

Yield: 5 cups

2 cups raw buckwheat groats

2 cups hempseeds

1 cup raw sunflower seeds

½ cup dates, pitted

½ cup water

¼ cup raw agave nectar

½ teaspoon sea salt

1 teaspoon ground cinnamon

¼ teaspoon grated nutmeg

This nutty crunchy granola is full of enzymes and a great way to get the good fats from hempseeds and sunflower seeds. You can add any fruit to this recipe; just remember to dehydrate for a few hours longer as fresh fruit has a higher water content. Dried fruit works very well, and the addition of Goji berries, an antioxidant-rich dried red berry from Tibet, will give this an extra nutritional punch. Once dehydrated, the granola will keep well in an airtight container for well over a week.

1. Rinse the buckwheat groats, then soak in 8 cups of water for 3 hours. Drain and rinse well in a colander until the water runs clear. Let sit for a few minutes, then pat dry with a clean towel.

2. Transfer the buckwheat groats to a large bowl and mix in the hempseeds and sunflower seeds.

3. In a blender, blend the dates and water together. Add the salt, agave nectar, cinnamon, and nutmeg; blend well.

4. Pour the spiced date mixture over the seed mixture and mix in.

5. Spread out thinly onto a Teflex dehydrating sheet and place in a dehydrator at 115°F for 12 hours, or until dry.

Bliss Cup

Serves 4

An impressive raw dessert that is both rich and healthful.

Carob Mousse

½ cup dates, pitted

1 cup water

1 tablespoon nonalcoholic
vanilla extract,
or ¼ vanilla bean,
scraped

3 ripe avocados, peeled,
pitted, and mashed

¾ cup carob powder, raw,
not roasted

¼ teaspoon sea salt

Vanilla-Cashew Cream

1 cup raw cashews

2 cups water

6 pitted dates, soaked
in ½ cup water

1 tablespoon nonalcoholic
vanilla extract, or
¼ vanilla bean, scraped

¼ teaspoon sea salt

Raspberry Topping

1 pint fresh raspberries, or
1 (10-ounce) bag frozen
raspberries, thawed

1 tablespoon agave syrup

Mint leaves, for garnish

Make the Mousse:

1. Soak the dates in the water for 20 minutes. Drain and set aside the soaking water.

2. In a food processor, blend the dates, vanilla, and salt until smooth. Add the avocados and process until smooth. Add the carob powder and 1 to 2 tablespoons of the date soaking water and blend until smooth.

Make the Cream:

1. Soak the cashews in the water for 20 minutes. Drain and discard the soaking water.

2. Combine the drained cashews, the dates and their soaking water, the vanilla extract, and the sea salt in a blender and blend until smooth.

Assemble the Bliss:

1. Spoon ½ cup of the mousse into the bottom of each of four sundae glasses or wineglasses.

2. Mix the raspberries with the agave nectar. Spoon ¼ cup of the raspberry mixture onto the mousse in each cup and top each with ¼ cup of the vanilla-cashew cream.

3. Repeat the procedure, layering the remaining mousse, berries, and vanilla-cashew cream, then garnish with fresh mint leaves and serve.

**TO SERVE: TOP WITH SOME
CHOPPED PECANS FOR ADDED CRUNCH!**

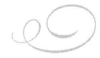

Nell's Coconut Rolls

Yield: 50 rolls

Our friend Nell loves anything with a tropical flair—
and these coconut date rolls are no exception. A simple, sweet,
decadent treat that is perfect for a bag lunch, picnic, or
as an afternoon pick-me-up snack.

8 ounces raw almonds,
about 1⅓ cups

½ teaspoon sea salt

1 tablespoon plus
1 teaspoon ground
cinnamon

2 cups pitted dates

2 tablespoons fresh lemon
juice

¼ cup coconut milk

1 cup unsweetened
shredded coconut

1. Process the almonds in a food processor to a sandy consistency and transfer to a medium-size bowl. Add the salt and 1 teaspoon of the cinnamon to the bowl and whisk to combine.

2. Process the dates in the food processor until smooth, scraping down the sides of the container as needed.

3. Add the processed dates, lemon juice, and coconut milk to the almond mixture and stir to combine.

4. Scoop the mixture out in teaspoons and roll into balls. Roll the balls in shredded coconut and sprinkle with the remaining cinnamon.

Raw Chocolates

Serves 6

This raw chocolate recipe will satisfy even the most dedicated chocoholic. Pure, simple, and rawsome!

1 cup raw cacao nibs
1 cup raw agave syrup
1½ cups coconut oil
Pinch of sea salt
½ cup finely chopped raw almonds

1. In a blender or food processor, blend all the ingredients except the almonds until completely smooth. Stir in the almonds.

2. Pour into candy molds or spread onto a sheet pan. Freeze until completely firm.

3. Store in the freezer until serving.

Raw Apple Pie

Yield: One 9-inch pie; serves 8

Guilt-free goodness even macrobiotic and diabetic people can enjoy. A filling of sliced apples, Medjool dates, and spices is piled high in a dehydrated pecan crust. Top with rich and creamy Raw Cream Whipped Topping.

1 cup Raw Cream
  Whipped Topping
  (page 167)

Raw Pecan Crust
2 cups pecans
2½ cups water
6 dates, pitted
1 tablespoon agave nectar, raw
1 tablespoon flaxseed oil
1 teaspoon ground cinnamon
½ teaspoon freshly ground nutmeg
1 tablespoon nonalcoholic vanilla extract
½ teaspoon sea salt

Lightly oil a 9-inch pie plate and set aside.

Make the Crust:

1. Soak the pecans in 2 cups of the water and the dates separately in ½ cup of water, for half an hour. Drain and rinse the nuts and fruit well.

2. In a food processor, chop the pecans into a fine meal and remove from the processor.

3. Put the soaked dates into the processor and chop. Add the chopped nuts, agave nectar, oil, spices, vanilla, and salt, and process until the mixture is sticky enough to hold a shape when pressed, but not too wet.

4. Transfer the mixture to the prepared pie plate and press the crust evenly up to the rim of the plate.

5. If a crisper crust is desired, dehydrate at 115°F for approximately 6 hours.

Make the Filling:

1. Soak the dates in the 3 cups of water for 30 to 40 minutes, or until soft. Drain, reserving the soaking water.

2. In a food processor, blend the dates using the soaking water as needed to produce a smooth mixture.

3. Pour the date mixture into a large mixing bowl. Add the apples, nutmeg, cinnamon, raisins, and lemon zest and juice, and mix well.

4. Fill the piecrust with the filling and chill. Serve with Raw Cream Whipped Topping.

Apple Filling

8 pitted dates

3 cups water

4 medium-size apples, peeled, cored, and sliced thinly

⅛ teaspoon nutmeg

½ teaspoon ground cinnamon

¼ cup raisins

Zest and juice of 1 lemon

Raw Cream Whipped Topping

A rich and smooth sweet topper for all your topping needs.

1 cup raw cashews

3 cups water

6 soft pitted dates

1 tablespoon raw agave nectar

2 tablespoons extra-virgin olive oil

1 tablespoon nonalcoholic vanilla extract

¼ teaspoon sea salt

1. Soak the cashews in 2 cups of the water for 30 to 40 minutes. Drain and rinse well.

2. Soak the dates in the remaining 1 cup of water until soft. Drain and reserve the soaking water.

3. Place the cashews, dates, agave nectar, oil, vanilla, and salt in a blender and blend, adding the date soaking water as needed until a smooth tahini-like consistency has been achieved.

Raw Lemon Pie

Yield: One 9-inch pie; serves 8

The rich blend of cashews, agave syrup, and fresh lemon juice will satisfy your sweet cravings without all of the refined sugars. Enjoy topped with fresh fruit for an extra treat.

Raw Brazil Nut Crust
1 cup Brazil nuts

2½ cups water

3 dried pineapple rings

6 pitted dates

1 cup coconut flakes

1 tablespoon raw
   agave nectar

1 tablespoon flaxseed oil

1 tablespoon ground
   cinnamon

1 teaspoon freshly ground
   nutmeg

1 tablespoon nonalcoholic
   vanilla extract

½ teaspoon sea salt

Lemon Cream Filling
2 cups raw cashews

7 cups water

1 cup pitted dates

½ teaspoon sea salt

¼ cup raw agave nectar

¼ cup fresh lemon juice

2 tablespoons nonalcoholic
   vanilla extract

Lightly oil a 9-inch pie plate and set aside.

Make the Piecrust:

1. Soak the Brazil nuts in 1 cup of water, the pineapple rings separately in 1 cup of water, and the dates in the remaining ½ cup of water for half an hour. Drain all and rinse well.

2. Place the drained nuts in a food processor, and process into a fine meal. Remove from the processor.

3. Put the soaked pineapple, dates, and coconut into the processor and chop. Add the chopped nuts, agave nectar, oil, spices, vanilla, and salt; mix well. The mixture should be sticky enough to hold its shape when pressed, but not too wet.

4. Press the crust evenly into the pie plate up to the rim.

5. If a crisper crust is desired, dehydrate at 115°F for approximately 6 hours.

Make the Filling:

1. Soak the cashews in 3 cups of water for half an hour. Drain and repeat with another 3 cups of water for another half hour, and drain again. Rinse well.

2. Soak the dates in the remaining 1 cup of water for 20 minutes. Drain, reserving the date soaking liquid, and rinse well.

3. Combine all the filling ingredients in a blender or food processor and blend well. Scrape down the sides as needed until smooth and creamy. Add the date soaking water as necessary.

4. Fill the piecrust with the filling and chill in the refrigerator to set.

Desserts

Mention "vegan desserts" and some people think of boring cookies that taste like sawdust. Not so with these gourmet goodies. One taste and even the most hard-to-convince sweet tooth will be won over. From our luscious Chocolate Ganache Cake to the holiday favorite Pumpkin Cheesecake, these desserts are easy to make, delicious, and wonderful to share for any occasion. Here you'll find a variety of treats, from our wildly popular Magic Cookie—a crunchy, chewy confection that's almost a meal unto itself—to the classic Tiramisu.

We use egg-free leaveners, healthier fats, and natural and alternative sweeteners, and recommend organic and more sustainable preparations of cane sugar to make these treats a little less harmful for you and the Earth—while not sacrificing taste, texture, or variety.

Hempseed–
Chocolate Chip Cookies

Yield: 16 cookies

Not just chocolate chip. These cookies are made from spelt flour and have the added bonus of hempseeds to make them healthy, as well as delicious.

2 cups spelt flour

½ teaspoon baking powder

1½ teaspoons egg replacer

¼ cup plus 2 tablespoons plus 2 more tablespoons water

¼ cup Sucanat

½ cup Florida Crystals

⅛ cup plus 1 tablespoon solid coconut oil

1 teaspoon vanilla extract

½ teaspoon salt

¼ cup vegan chocolate chips

2 tablespoons hempseeds

1. Combine the spelt flour and baking powder in a large bowl. Set aside.

2. In a separate bowl, whisk together the egg replacer and 2 tablespoons of the water. Add the Sucanat, Florida Crystals, and coconut oil, and cream well by hand or with an electric mixer. Stir in the vanilla and salt.

3. Mix the wet ingredients into the dry. Stir in the chocolate chips and hempseeds.

4. Stir in the remaining ¼ cup plus 2 tablespoons of water slowly, and then let the dough chill for 20 minutes.

5. Preheat the oven to 350°F. Line a large baking sheet with baking parchment.

6. Scoop the batter into golf ball–size balls. Space 2 inches apart on the prepared baking sheet.

7. Bake for approximately 18 minutes, until golden brown. Remove from the oven and let cool on the baking sheet.

Jam Dot Cookies (Peanut Butter and Jam Cookies)

Yield: 14 large cookies

Dry Ingredients

2½ cups roasted salted peanuts

2½ cups rolled oats

2½ cups spelt flour

Pinch of sea salt

1½ teaspoons ground cinnamon

Wet Ingredients

1¼ cups maple syrup

1¼ cups canola oil

Raspberry fruit spread, for filling

Preheat the oven to 350°F. Line a large baking sheet with baking parchment.

1. Pulse the peanuts in a food processor or blender to a medium grind. Transfer to a medium-size bowl. Pulse the oats until finely ground, and add to the bowl containing the ground peanuts. Add the flour, salt, and cinnamon to the bowl, and stir to combine.

2. In a second medium-size bowl, combine the wet ingredients.

3. Add the wet ingredients to the dry and mix until combined.

4. Scoop ¼-cup mounds of dough onto the prepared baking sheet. Space 2 inches apart and flatten with your palm. Indent the middle of each cookie and fill with about 1 tablespoon of the fruit spread.

5. Bake for 15 to 20 minutes until golden. Remove from the oven and let cool on the baking sheet.

CHEF'S TIP: A DEEPER WELL ENSURES THAT THE JAM DOES NOT BUBBLE OVER DURING BAKING.

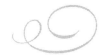

Magic Cookies

Yield: 9 large cookies

These cookies—a combination of coconut, carrots, pecans, and chocolate chips baked until golden brown—make magic happen.

⅓ cup vegan chocolate chips

2 cups pecans, chopped

Dry Ingredients

1 cup unbleached all-purpose flour

¾ cup shredded carrots

1 cup coconut

1 cup Florida Crystals

1 cup rolled oats

½ teaspoon baking powder

¼ teaspoon salt

Wet Ingredients

2 tablespoons coconut oil, melted

⅓ cup water

¼ cup canola oil

1½ teaspoons vanilla extract

Preheat the oven to 350°F. Line a large baking sheet with baking parchment.

1. In a large bowl, mix together the flour, carrots, coconut, Florida Crystals, oats, baking powder, and salt.

2. In a separate bowl, mix together the coconut oil, water, canola oil, and vanilla.

3. Add the wet ingredients to the dry, and mix well to combine. Stir in the chocolate chips and pecans.

4. Scoop ¼-cup mounds of dough onto the prepared baking sheet. Space 2 inches apart and flatten with your palm.

5. Bake for 10 to 15 minutes, until golden brown. Remove from the oven and let cool on the baking sheet.

Maple-Pecan Cookies

Yield: 12 large cookies

A delicious treat on its own with tea or coffee, we also use this basic cookie for our cheesecake crust (see page 181). It contains no refined sugar.

Pecan halves, for garnish

Wet Ingredients

1 cup canola oil

1 cup maple syrup

2 tablespoons vanilla extract

¼ teaspoon salt

Dry Ingredients

3 cups pecans, toasted and ground

2 cups rolled oats

2 cups spelt flour

Preheat the oven to 350°F. Line a large baking sheet with baking parchment.

1. In a medium-size bowl, combine the oil, maple syrup, vanilla, and salt.

2. Pulse the pecans in a food processor or blender to a medium grind. Transfer to a medium-size bowl. Pulse the oats until finely ground, and add them to the bowl with the ground pecans. Add the spelt flour to the bowl, and stir to combine.

3. Add the wet ingredients to the dry, and mix thoroughly.

4. Scoop ¼-cup mounds of dough onto the prepared baking sheet. Space 2 inches apart and flatten with your palm.

5. Bake for 20 minutes until golden. Remove from the oven and let cool on the baking sheet.

Oatmeal-Raisin Cookies

Yield: 12 large cookies

These cookies are an old-fashioned standby, but never fail to bring joy and smiles to the mouths of those who eat them.

3 teaspoons egg replacer
1¼ cups water
1 cup coconut oil
1½ cups Florida Crystals
1½ cups Sucanat
2 teaspoons vanilla extract
6 tablespoons soy milk

1 cup canola oil
4½ cups unbleached
   all-purpose flour
1 teaspoon baking powder
1 teaspoon salt
2½ cups rolled oats
2 teaspoons ground
   cinnamon
1 teaspoon grated nutmeg
¼ teaspoon ground ginger
1 cup raisins
½ cup chopped walnuts

Preheat the oven to 350°F. Line a large baking sheet with baking parchment.

1. In a medium-size bowl, whisk together the egg replacer and ¼ cup of the water. Add the coconut oil, Florida Crystals, and Sucanat, and cream together. Add the vanilla, soy milk, oil, and remaining water, and mix well.

2. In a separate bowl, stir together the flour, baking powder, salt, oats, cinnamon, nutmeg, and ginger.

3. Add the dry ingredients to the wet, and mix well. Stir in the raisins and walnuts.

4. Scoop ¼-cup mounds of dough onto the baking sheet. Space 2 inches apart and flatten with your palm.

5. Bake for 15 to 18 minutes. Remove from the oven and let cool on the baking sheet.

Sugar Cookies

Yield: 12 large cookies

Dry Ingredients

4½ cups spelt flour

¾ teaspoon baking soda

½ teaspoon salt

½ teaspoon ground cinnamon

Wet Ingredients

3 tablespoons egg replacer

¾ cup water

2¼ cups Florida Crystals

1 tablespoon vanilla extract

1 cup plus 2 tablespoons canola or other flavorless oil

2 tablespoons maple syrup

These crisp cookies are easy and fabulous to make around the holidays. If chilled, they can be rolled out, cut, and decorated like traditional butter sugar cookies.

Preheat the oven to 350°F. Line a large baking sheet with baking parchment.

1. Sift the flour, baking soda, salt, and cinnamon together into a large bowl.

2. In a separate bowl, whisk together the egg replacer and the water, then mix in the Florida Crystals, vanilla, oil, and maple syrup.

3. Pour the wet ingredients into the dry, and mix together thoroughly.

4. Roll into ¼-cup balls, space 2 inches apart on the prepared baking sheet, and flatten with your palm.

5. Bake for 15 to 18 minutes, or until golden. Remove from the oven and let cool on the baking sheet.

VARIATION: GINGER SPICE COOKIES:
REPLACE THE MAPLE SYRUP WITH MOLASSES,
AND ADD 2 TEASPOONS OF GROUND GINGER,
1 TEASPOON OF GROUND CINNAMON, ½ TEASPOON
OF GRATED NUTMEG, AND 1 TEASPOON OF ALLSPICE.

Desserts

Lacy Sesame-Almond Cookies

Yield: 24 cookies

These cookies are crispy and pretty. Serve them with any nondairy frozen confection or eat them alone.

7 tablespoons vegan margarine

1 cup Sucanat

1 tablespoon maple syrup

1 tablespoon vanilla extract

1 cup rolled oats

3 tablespoons sesame seeds

¼ cup toasted almond slivers

3 tablespoons unbleached all-purpose flour

Pinch of sea salt

1. Blend all the ingredients in a food processor until well blended.

2. Refrigerate the dough and let chill for at least half an hour.

3. About 10 minutes before the dough is done chilling, preheat the oven to 400°F. Line two baking sheets with baking parchment.

4. Roll the chilled dough by tablespoons into balls and place far apart on the prepared baking sheets, keeping the remaining dough chilled in the refrigerator between batches. About six cookies may be baked per sheet.

5. Bake the cookies until they spread to look like lace—8 to 10 minutes. Let cool completely before removing from the baking sheet. When these cookies cool enough to touch, you can wrap them around a wooden spoon handle or press them into a mini-cupcake pan to make a cup shape, either of which can be filled with any of your favorite fillings.

Blondies

Yield: 9 blondies

2 tablespoons tahini

1 tablespoon peanut butter

1 cup vegan chocolate chips

Dry Ingredients

1 cup whole wheat flour

1 cup plus 6 tablespoons unbleached all-purpose flour

1 teaspoon baking powder

1 teaspoon salt

Wet Ingredients

½ cup Sucanat

½ cup finely ground coffee

1 cup canola oil

1 cup maple syrup

½ cup soy milk

¼ cup vanilla extract

Coffee, chocolate, peanut butter, and maple syrup combine to make these four-star blondies a winner with everyone. For a caffeine-free treat, leave out the coffee, or use decaffeinated coffee.

Preheat the oven to 350°F. Line the bottom of an 8-inch square pan with baking parchment.

1. Sift the dry ingredients together into a large mixing bowl.

2. In a separate bowl, mix together the Sucanat, ground coffee, oil, maple syrup, soy milk, and vanilla.

3. Add the wet ingredients to the dry and mix until moistened. Stir in the tahini and peanut butter, then stir in the chocolate chips.

4. Spread the batter into the prepared baking pan and bake for 18 minutes, or until a toothpick inserted into the center comes out clean. Remove from the oven and let cool in the pan on a rack to room temperature. Cut into nine equal squares.

Desserts

Brownies

Yield: 24 large brownies (recipe can easily be halved)

Super-rich chocolaty goodness, these brownies beg to be eaten with a tall glass of your favorite soy or nut milk. Spread chocolate ganache on top of them to drive your friends and family into a chocoholic frenzy.

Preheat the oven to 350°F. Grease a 9 by 13-inch pan and line with baking parchment.

1. Whisk together the water and the egg replacer, and then mix with the rest of the wet ingredients and Sucanat.

2. In a separate bowl, stir together the cocoa, flour, baking powder, salt, and nuts.

3. Add the wet ingredients to the dry and mix together.

4. Pour into the prepared pan and bake for 25 to 30 minutes, or until a toothpick inserted into the center comes out clean. Cool on a rack to room temperature. When cool, cut into twenty-four squares.

Wet Ingredients

3 tablespoons egg replacer

¾ cup water

1½ cups soy milk

1¼ cups oil

1 tablespoon vanilla extract

3 cups Sucanat

Dry Ingredients

2¼ cups unsweetened cocoa powder

2 cups unbleached all-purpose flour

¾ teaspoon baking powder

¾ teaspoon salt

1½ cups chopped nuts

Elise's Apple Crisp

Serves 8–12

Filling
5 pounds Braeburn apples, peeled, cored, and sliced

3 tablespoons lemon juice

¼ teaspoon sea salt

½ cup evaporated cane juice

1 teaspoon ground ginger

½ teaspoon grated nutmeg

3 tablespoons arrowroot powder

Topping
2 cups spelt flour

2 cups rolled oats

½ teaspoon sea salt

½ cup evaporated cane juice

1 tablespoon ground cinnamon

¾ cup sunflower oil

**TO SERVE:
TOP WITH VANILLA SOY.
DELICIOUS FOR AN
EXTRA-SPECIAL TREAT.**

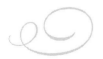

Our friend Elise Spiro has created many delicious desserts, this crisp being a favorite. She says, "I love making this recipe for potlucks; it's fast, easy, and serves a lot of people. During different times of year I love substituting the apples for different seasonal fruit like strawberry-rhubarb, peaches, or pears."

Preheat the oven to 350°F.

Make the Filling:

1. In a medium-size bowl, combine the apples, lemon juice, salt, cane juice, ginger, nutmeg, and arrowroot. Mix well. Spread evenly in a 9 by 13-inch baking dish.

Make the Topping:

1. In another bowl, stir together the spelt flour, oats, salt, cane juice, and cinnamon. Drizzle in ¾ cup of the oil.

2. Mix together with a spoon or use your hands to form crumbs. Add up to an extra ¼ cup of oil if needed. Sprinkle evenly over the filling.

3. Bake for 40 to 45 minutes, or until the crisp starts bubbling and the topping is golden brown. Let cool a little before serving. Serve warm or cool.

**VARIATIONS:
OMIT 1 APPLE AND ADD
1 CUP OF BERRIES TO THE FILLING, AND ADD ½ CUP OF YOUR
FAVORITE CHOPPED NUTS TO THE TOPPING.**

**FOR A STRAWBERRY-RHUBARB CRISP,
ADD 2 TEASPOONS OF LEMON ZEST AND OMIT THE NUTMEG.**

**FOR A PEACH CRISP, SUBSTITUTE 2 TEASPOONS OF
GRATED OR MINCED FRESH GINGER FOR THE
GROUND GINGER IN THE FILLING, AND OMIT THE NUTMEG;
AND ADD ½ CUP OF CHOPPED ALMONDS TO THE TOPPING.**

Pecan Bars

Yield: 12 bars

This recipe for buttery, crunchy pecan bars is easier to make than you would think.

Preheat the oven to 350°F.

Make the Crust:

1. In a small bowl, combine the flour, Sucanat, and cane juice. Add the melted vegan margarine and soy milk. Mix until combined.

2. Press the mixture into a 9 by 13-inch baking dish.

3. Prebake the crust for 10 minutes. Leaving the oven on, remove the crust from the oven and spread the pecans over the top.

Make the Topping:

1. In a small saucepan, combine the remaining Sucanat, margarine, and vanilla. Cook over low heat, stirring constantly, until the margarine is melted and the Sucanat is dissolved.

2. When the mixture comes to a slow simmer, continue stirring, and cook for an additional minute. Pour the mixture evenly over the crust and pecans.

3. Return the bars to the oven and bake for 15 to 20 minutes, until the topping is golden and bubbly. Let cool completely before cutting and serving.

Crust
4 cups whole wheat pastry flour

½ cup Sucanat

1 cup evaporated cane juice

1 cup melted vegan margarine

⅓ cup soy milk

Topping
3 cups pecans

1 cup Sucanat

1½ cups vegan margarine

1 tablespoon vanilla extract

Cheesecake

Yield: One 9-inch cake; serves 8

This tofu cheesecake is wheat free, cholesterol free, and as creamy and delicious as what your Mom used to make.

Preheat the oven to 375°F. Grease a 9-inch springform pan.

Fruit Sauce
(recipe follows)

Crust

1 cup rolled oats,
  ground finely
1½ cups pecans, toasted
  and finely ground
1 cup spelt flour
½ cup canola oil
½ cup maple syrup
1 tablespoon vanilla extract
⅛ teaspoon sea salt

Filling

2 (14-ounce) blocks
  extra-firm tofu
½ cup canola oil
½ teaspoon sea salt
¼ cup lemon juice
1 cup Florida Crystals
1 tablespoon vanilla extract

Make the Crust:

1. Combine the oats, pecans, and spelt flour in a mixing bowl.

2. In a separate bowl, combine the oil, maple syrup, vanilla, and salt.

3. Mix the wet ingredients into the dry and press into the prepared pan. Bake for 10 minutes, then remove from the oven and set aside.

Make the Filling:

1. Combine the ingredients for the filling in a blender or food processor, and blend until smooth.

Assemble the Cheesecake:

1. Pour the filling into the crust and bake for 25 minutes.

2. Remove from the oven and let cool to room temperature in the pan. Refrigerate for 1 hour before serving. Serve with Fruit Sauce.

Desserts

Fruit Sauce

Yield: 2 cups

This sauce is sweet and delicious. Try it over ice cream or with our Cheesecake or Chocolate Ganache Cake (see page 185).

3 cups fresh or frozen fruit of choice

3 tablespoons lemon juice

¼ cup arrowroot powder

¼ cup cold water

½ cup Florida Crystals

Pinch of sea salt

1. In a small saucepan, combine the fruit, lemon juice, and Florida Crystals, and heat over medium-low heat. Cook for 3 to 4 minutes, stirring until the crystals dissolve.

2. Dissolve the arrowroot in cold water, stirring well to be sure it makes a cloudy liquid with no powder settled on the bottom.

3. Add the arrowroot mixture to the fruit in the pot, stirring continuously to avoid lumps. Add a pinch of salt and cook for 3 to 5 minutes, stirring, until thickened.

4. Let the sauce cool. Store in the refrigerator for up to 3 days.

CHEF'S TIP: FOR A THINNER SAUCE, REMOVE THE SAUCE FROM THE HEAT BEFORE ADDING THE ARROWROOT, ADD A PINCH OF SALT, LET COOL, AND BLEND. POUR THE MIXTURE THROUGH A SIEVE AND YOU WILL HAVE A SMOOTH AND REFINED SAUCE.

Pumpkin Cheesecake

Yield: One 9-inch cake; serves 8

Pumpkin cheesecake is a holiday classic flavored with the sweet spices of autumn—cinnamon, nutmeg, and ginger. The pecan crust adds the final touch to make this pie part of your family's holiday tradition.

Pecan Cookie Crust

1 cup rolled oats, ground finely

1½ cups pecans, toasted and ground finely

1 cup whole wheat pastry flour

½ cup canola oil

½ cup maple syrup

1 tablespoon vanilla extract

⅛ teaspoon sea salt

Pumpkin Filling

2 cups pumpkin puree, or 1 (15-ounce) can

1 (14-ounce) block extra-firm tofu

½ cup safflower oil

¼ teaspoon salt

¼ cup maple syrup

1 cup Sucanat

1 tablespoon vanilla extract

¾ teaspoon ground cinnamon

¼ teaspoon grated nutmeg

½ teaspoon ground ginger

CHEF'S TIP:
ALWAYS TURN OFF YOUR BLENDER BEFORE SCRAPING THE SIDES.

Preheat the oven to 350°F.

Make the Crust:

1. Combine the oats, pecans, and pastry flour in a mixing bowl.

2. In a separate bowl, combine the canola oil, maple syrup, vanilla, and salt.

3. Stir the wet ingredients into the dry and press into a 9-inch springform pan to form a crust.

Make the Filling:

1. Combine all of the filling ingredients in a blender or food processor, and process until smooth, pausing to scrape down the sides of the container with a spatula as you go.

Assemble the Cheesecake:

1. Pour the filling into the prepared crust. Bake for 30 minutes.

2. Remove from the oven and cool on a rack to room temperature. Cover and chill for 4 hours before serving.

Chocolate Cake

Yield: Two 9-inch layers; serves 8

These basic chocolate layers are the starting point

for many of the cakes that follow.

Dry Ingredients
2 cups unbleached all-purpose flour
½ cup unsweetened cocoa powder
½ cup Sucanat
2 teaspoons baking powder
2 teaspoons baking soda
1 teaspoon salt

Wet Ingredients
½ cup canola oil
1 cup vanilla soy milk
½ cup water
1 cup maple syrup
1 tablespoon chocolate extract
2 teaspoons apple cider vinegar

Preheat the oven to 350°F. Oil two 9-inch round cake pans and set aside.

1. Sift the flour, cocoa, Sucanat, baking powder, baking soda, and salt into a large bowl and stir together.

2. In a separate bowl, mix together the oil, soy milk, water, maple syrup, chocolate extract, and vinegar.

3. Pour the wet ingredients into the dry and stir until incorporated.

4. Divide the batter evenly between the two prepared pans, and bake for 18 to 22 minutes, until a toothpick inserted into the center of the cake comes out clean. Cool the layers in their pans on racks for 10 minutes, then remove from the pans. Cool to room temperature on the racks before frosting.

Chocolate Ganache Cake

Yield: One 9-inch cake; serves 8

Chocolate Ganache
Yield: 1 pint

2 cups vegan chocolate chips

1 cup vanilla soy milk

1 recipe Chocolate Cake (2 layers), baked and cooled (page 184)

TO SERVE:
SERVE DRIZZLED WITH CHOCOLATE SAUCE (RECIPE FOLLOWS) FOR A CHOCOHOLIC DELIGHT.

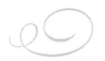

On our restaurant's menu every week since we opened our doors, this decadent chocolate fantasy put us on the map for top-notch vegan desserts. We now gladly pass it on to you to enjoy!

1. Put the chocolate chips in a medium-size heatproof bowl.

2. Slowly heat the soy milk to the boiling point. Pour over the chips and let sit for 1 to 2 minutes, until the chocolate is softened. Whisk the chips and milk together well for about 2 minutes, until the frosting takes on a velvety gloss.

3. Chill for at least 1½ hours, until solid.

4. Frost the cake: place one layer on a cake plate, frost the top with a ½-inch layer of frosting, then top with the second layer. Frost the sides and then the top of the entire cake.

Chocolate Sauce

Yield: 1 pint

1 cup vegan chocolate chips

2 cups vanilla soy milk

This recipe makes a thin, rich chocolate sauce that is a fitting accompaniment to many desserts.

Follow the directions for the Chocolate Ganache Cake through step 3.

TO SERVE:
TRY THIS DRIZZLED OVER CAKE OR ICE CREAM—ANYWHERE A FESTIVE FINISH IS DESIRED.

Desserts

German Chocolate Cake

Yield: One 9-inch cake; serves 8

The toasted pecans and coconut in this topping for our basic chocolate cake take it to another level of indulgence.

1 recipe Chocolate Cake (2 layers), baked and cooled (page 184)

Coconut Frosting
¼ cup egg replacer
1 cup water
⅔ cup coconut milk
2 cups Sucanat
¼ cup coconut oil
1½ cups toasted coconut
1¼ cups chopped pecans
1 teaspoon coconut extract
Pinch of nutmeg
½ teaspoon vanilla extract
1 teaspoon sea salt

1. In a small saucepan, whisk together the egg replacer, water, coconut milk, and Sucanat until well incorporated.

2. Cook over medium-low heat for 3 minutes. Add the coconut oil, toasted coconut, pecans, coconut extract, and nutmeg, and continue to cook, stirring constantly, until the mixture has thickened slightly.

3. Add the vanilla and cook for about 2 minutes. Add the salt and cook until the mixture has darkened to an even shade of tan, stirring constantly.

4. Refrigerate the frosting until set, then use this frosting to fill the middle and frost the top of the cake. Use chocolate ganache for the sides of the cake.

Peanut Butter–Chocolate Cake

Yield: One 9-inch cake; serves 8

The winning combination of chocolate and peanut butter can't go wrong. Our rich chocolate cake frosted with this luscious whipped peanut butter frosting is a case in point.

1 recipe Chocolate Cake (2 layers), baked and cooled (page 184)

Peanut Butter Frosting
1 stick (½ cup) Earth Balance shortening
3½ cups confectioners' sugar
1½ teaspoons vanilla extract
¼ cup plain soy milk
½ cup creamy natural peanut butter

Make the Peanut Butter Frosting:
1. Place all the frosting ingredients in a food processor and blend until creamy.

Assemble the Cake:
1. Frost one layer of the cake with the peanut butter frosting, then top with the second layer and frost the sides and top with either peanut butter frosting or chocolate ganache.

TO SERVE: DRIZZLE THE PLATES WITH CHOCOLATE SAUCE (PAGE 185) FOR A DAZZLING FINISH!

186

Vanilla Cake

Yield: Two 9-inch layers

3½ cups unbleached
    all-purpose flour
2 teaspoons baking powder
2 teaspoons baking soda
1 teaspoon salt
⅔ cup canola oil
1½ cups maple syrup
1⅓ cups water
¼ cup vanilla extract
⅛ cup apple cider vinegar

This is a basic vanilla cake recipe that can be a great jumping-off point. Try frosting this with vanilla frosting or chocolate ganache, or use your imagination and have fun with this delicious base.

Preheat the oven to 350°F. Oil two 9-inch round pans and line with baking parchment.

1. In a large bowl, sift together the flour, baking powder, baking soda, and salt.

2. In a medium-size bowl, combine the oil, maple syrup, water, vanilla, and vinegar.

3. Pour the wet ingredients into the dry and mix until combined. Divide the batter evenly between the prepared pans.

4. Bake for approximately 20 minutes, until the tops are golden and a toothpick inserted into the center comes out clean. Cool the layers on a rack for 10 minutes and remove from the pans. Let cool on the racks to room temperature before frosting.

CHEF'S TIP: USING BOTH OIL AND BAKING PARCHMENT TO LINE THE CAKE PANS ENSURES THAT THE CAKE RELEASES CLEANLY FROM THE BOTTOM OF THE PAN. WHEN THE LAYERS HAVE COOLED FOR 10 MINUTES, RUN A THIN KNIFE AROUND THE OUTSIDE EDGE OF THE PAN AND INVERT THE CAKE ONTO A HEATPROOF PLATE OR EXTRA BAKING RACK. THEN PEEL THE PARCHMENT OFF THE CAKE. VOILÀ! CLEAN FINISH EVERY TIME. COMPLETE THE COOLING ON RACKS.

Vanilla Frosting

Yield: Approximately 4 cups

This recipe makes enough to frost and fill a 9-inch two-layer cake.

1½ cups Florida Crystals

2 teaspoons agar

1½ tablespoons water

2 (14-ounce) blocks
firm tofu

½ cup coconut oil

½ cup canola oil

¼ cup maple syrup

½ teaspoon salt

1 tablespoon vanilla extract

1. Put the Florida Crystals, agar, and water into a small saucepan. Stir to dissolve and cook over medium heat until syrupy.

2. Process the tofu, coconut oil, canola oil, maple syrup, salt, and vanilla in a blender.

3. Add the syrupy mixture to the mixture in the blender and blend until smooth. Refrigerate overnight.

Lemon-Coconut Cake

Yield: One 9-inch cake; serves 8

Layers of cake are filled with tart lemon curd, frosted with our creamy vanilla-coconut frosting, and topped with coconut curls. This cake will make a beautiful addition to a garden party or anytime tea.

1 recipe Vanilla Cake
(2 layers), baked and
cooled (page 187)

Vanilla-Coconut Frosting
(page 189)

½ cup untoasted coconut
flakes

1 cup toasted coconut

Lemon Curd Filling

2 cups apple cider

⅛ teaspoon turmeric

2½ tablespoons agar

1 cup rice syrup

¼ cup maple syrup

¾ cup lemon juice

¼ cup arrowroot powder

½ cup soy milk

4 teaspoons lemon zest

Pinch of salt

2 teaspoons vanilla extract

Make the Lemon Curd Filling:

1. In a medium-size saucepan, combine all the curd filling ingredients, and cook over medium-low heat, stirring, until mixture starts to thicken, about 10 minutes.

2. Chill for at least 4 hours, and then stir again to reach a spreadable consistency.

Assemble the Cake:

1. Level each cake by slicing off any rounded top. Then slice each cake in half horizontally to make four equal layers.

2. Spread ¾ cup of lemon curd evenly onto one layer of the cake. Drop 3 tablespoons of the Vanilla-Coconut Frosting onto the center of the layer.

3. Top with a second layer, and repeat step 2. Repeat with the third layer. Place the fourth layer on top.

4. Frost the outside of the cake with the remaining frosting. Sprinkle the coconut on the cake to finish.

CHEF'S TIP: THE VANILLA-COCONUT FROSTING SHOULD BE REFRIGERATED OVERNIGHT, SO BE SURE TO MAKE IT IN ADVANCE.

Rain Forest Crunch Cake

Yield: One 9-inch cake; serves 8

This moist, rich banana cake layered with chocolate ganache and fluffy vanilla-coconut frosting is coated with a delightful blend of sweet and crunchy Brazil nuts.

1 recipe Vanilla Cake (2 layers) made with banana (instructions follow), baked and cooled (page 187)

chocolate ganache (page 185)

Vanilla-Coconut Frosting

½ cup coconut oil

1 cup coconut milk

¼ cup maple syrup

1½ teaspoons sea salt

1½ cups organic sugar

1 tablespoon vanilla extract

2 (14-ounce) blocks extra-firm tofu, crumbled

2 cups vegan chocolate chips

1 cup vanilla soy milk

Brazil Nut Crunch

3 cups chopped Brazil nuts

½ cup maple syrup

½ cup Florida Crystals

½ teaspoon sea salt

Make the Vanilla-Coconut Frosting:

1. In a blender, blend the coconut oil, coconut milk, maple syrup, sea salt, sugar, and vanilla until mixed.

2. With the blender running on low speed, slowly add the crumbled tofu. Replace the lid and blend until smooth and glossy, scraping down the sides of the container a couple times.

3. Refrigerate overnight.

Make the Banana Cake:

1. Prepare the Vanilla Cake with the addition of one large ripe banana, mashed, mixed into the wet ingredients.

Make the Brazil Nut Crunch:

Preheat the oven to 375°F. Line a baking sheet with baking parchment and brush with a light coating of canola oil.

1. In a bowl, mix all the ingredients well until the sugar starts to dissolve.

2. Spread the mixture in the center of the prepared baking sheet and bake for 5 minutes. Turn the sheet around front to back and bake for an additional 5 minutes.

3. Remove the sheet from the oven and let the Brazil Nut Crunch cool until hard and brittle. Pull up the parchment and gently break up the brittle.

4. Transfer the brittle to a food processor and pulse to a rough, gravel-like consistency—we like some pieces crumb size and others larger. Set aside.

Assemble the Cake:

1. Place one of the cooled cake layers on a plate, and spread the top with the chocolate ganache.

2. Carefully place the second layer on top of the first, checking to make sure they're lined up. Frost the top and the sides of the cake with the Vanilla-Coconut Frosting.

3. Using your hand as a scoop, press the Brazil Nut Crunch into the frosted sides of the cake.

Tiramisu

Yield: 12 squares

This traditional Italian classic is a rich and creamy perennial favorite—even without dairy or eggs.

1 recipe Vanilla Cake, baked as a single layer in a jelly roll pan (page 187)

Vanilla Frosting (page 188)

½ cup prepared strong coffee or espresso

1 cup chopped vegan chocolate chips

To Assemble the Tiramisu:

1. Cut the cake in half widthwise and place one-half in the bottom of a 9 by 13-inch baking dish.

2. Moisten the cake with the coffee, then top with 1½ cups of the vanilla frosting. Sprinkle with ½ cup of the chocolate chips.

3. Place the other half of the cake on top, and then spread the remaining vanilla frosting evenly over the cake. Sprinkle with the remaining chocolate chips.

4. Cover and refrigerate to let set, and then slice into squares and serve.

Luscious Chocolate Brownie–Hazelnut Mousse Torte

Yield: One 9-inch cake; serves 8

Chocolate and hazelnuts is a famous pairing of flavors but usually involves dairy. This torte tastes so rich that no one will believe it's vegan.

Preheat the oven to 350°F. Oil a 9-inch springform pan.

Make the Brownie Crust:

1. In a medium-size bowl, combine the oil, maple syrup, soy milk, and vanilla, and whisk to combine.

2. In a large bowl, stir together all the dry ingredients except the chocolate chips.

3. Fold the wet ingredients into the dry and gently mix. Fold in the chocolate chips.

4. Pour the batter into the oiled pan and bake for 20 to 25 minutes. Remove from the oven to cool on a rack.

Make the Chocolate-Hazelnut Mousse:

1. While the crust is cooling, melt the chocolate chips in the top part of a double boiler over boiling water.

2. Place the remaining mousse ingredients in a blender or food processor, and process until smooth. With the machine still running, add the melted chocolate.

3. Pour the mousse over the cooled brownie crust. Return the pan to the oven and bake for another 15 to 20 minutes, or until the mousse pulls away from the sides of the pan.

4. Let the torte cool to the touch, cover, and refrigerate for 2 hours until completely firm.

Brownie Crust

½ cup canola oil

½ cup maple syrup

¼ cup soy milk

1½ teaspoons vanilla extract

1 cup unbleached all-purpose flour

½ cup unsweetened cocoa powder

6 tablespoons Florida Crystals

¼ cup Sucanat

1 teaspoon baking powder

¾ teaspoon sea salt

½ cup vegan chocolate chips

Chocolate-Hazelnut Mousse

1 cup vegan chocolate chips

1 (12.3-ounce) package firm or extra-firm silken lite tofu

6 tablespoons Sucanat

½ teaspoon vanilla extract

Pinch of sea salt

1½ teaspoons chocolate extract

2 tablespoons hazelnut butter or any nut butter you like

Kit's Peach Skillet Cobbler

Serves 4–6

3 tablespoons coconut oil
1 tablespoon apricot butter or all-fruit preserves
4 pounds peaches, skinned, pitted, and sliced (about 8 medium-size peaches)
¾ cup plus 2 tablespoons Sucanat
1 tablespoon lemon juice
1 cup unbleached all-purpose flour
2 teaspoons baking powder
¼ teaspoon salt
¾ cup soy milk or other nondairy milk

This is our friend Kit's vegan adaptation of a simple classic. The recipe works best with a 12-inch cast-iron skillet, but any oven-safe skillet or stove-to-oven 2-quart casserole will do.

Preheat the oven to 400°F.

1. Melt the coconut oil in a 12-inch cast-iron skillet over medium-high heat and stir in the apricot butter.

2. Add the sliced peaches, 2 tablespoons of the Sucanat, and the lemon juice, and stir until the fruit softens a bit, 3 to 5 minutes.

3. In a medium-size bowl, mix together the flour, baking powder, remaining Sucanat, and salt. Stir in the soy milk to make a batter.

4. Spoon the batter evenly over the fruit in the skillet. Transfer the skillet to the oven and bake for 25 minutes, until the cobbler is golden brown. Serve warm.

CHEF'S TIP:
TO SKIN PEACHES, SCORE THE BOTTOM OF EACH PEACH WITH A SHALLOW X.
DROP THE PEACHES INTO BOILING WATER FOR 30 SECONDS, THEN IMMEDIATELY TRANSFER THEM TO A BOWL OF COLD WATER. THE SKINS WILL NOW EASILY PEEL RIGHT OFF.

TO SERVE: FOR AN EXTRA TREAT,
SERVE WITH A SCOOP OF VANILLA SOY—DELICIOUS!

VARIATIONS: YOU CAN EASILY ADAPT THIS RECIPE FOR EACH SEASON'S FRUIT HARVEST. SIMPLY REPLACE THE PEACH SLICES WITH 4–5 CUPS OF BERRIES, CHOPPED RHUBARB, SLICED APPLES, PEARS, STONE FRUIT, OR ANY COMBINATION OF THE ABOVE.

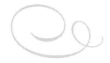

Kids' Food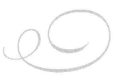

An early understanding of how food choices can be healthy, fun, and delicious, while still being Earth-friendly, is priceless knowledge for any child. This section offers some creative tips for starting kids off on a healthy path and provides some recipes designed just for them.

RAISING HEALTHY EATERS

Allow your children to develop a relationship with their food. Make food shopping an enjoyable experience by talking to your children as you shop, telling them where the food comes from and what it can do for their bodies. If you have the opportunity, take your children to the local farmers' market and let them meet the farmers who grow their food. Give them the chance to smell the food, touch it, and appreciate it. Allow them to choose—would you like an apple or a banana? But most of all, prepare the food for your child with love in your heart and try to eat smart. Children learn what they live.

FEEDING KIDS ON TRIPS

These are some simple ideas for food to bring on a long or short trip:

- Dried fruit
- Fruit leather
- Juice boxes
- Small boxes of soy milk
- Jars of all-natural vegan baby food

- Trail mix
- Bottled water
- Steamed vegetables
- Crackers and pretzels
- Strips of toasted nori

For special treats, have a few natural lollipops tucked away.

FAVORITE FINGER FOODS

- O-shaped cereals
- Rice cakes
- Well-cooked diced carrots
- Whole-grain toast with the crusts removed
- French toast
- Ripe pear slices
- Cooked apple slices

- Tofu chunks
- Cooked peas
- Cooked pasta
- Avocado chunks

"BE WARY" FOODS

The foods listed below can be a choking hazard for tiny throats. Most of these foods are suitable for children over one year of age, but keep a watch on your toddler when these items are served.

- Nuts
- Seeds
- Raw carrots
- Grapes
- Popcorn
- Celery
- Raw apples

Ants on a Log

Munch away on these little snacks.

Celery stalks
Nut butter of choice
Raisins

1. Cut the celery into three pieces and fill with the nut butter. Top with raisins and enjoy.

VARIATION: BLOB ON A BISCUIT: USE CRACKERS INSTEAD OF CELERY, AND JAM OR JELLY INSTEAD OF RAISINS.

Baby's Apricot-Apple Puree

You can alter this recipe to your baby's tastes by substituting an equal amount of pears, peaches, or just about any fruit for the apples and/or apricots.

2 medium-size apples, peeled, cored, and chopped
6 dried apricots, chopped finely
Water

1. Place the apples and apricots in a pan with just enough water to cover. Bring to a boil, turn down the heat, and simmer for 5 minutes.
2. Drain the fruit, reserving the cooking liquid.
3. Puree the fruit mixture with a blender or hand blender, adding the reserved cooking water to thin if desired.

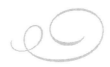

Baby's Hot Cereals

Serves 1

Banana Hot Cereal

1 tablespoon uncooked rolled oats

¾ cup water

1 small banana

2 teaspoons golden raisins

Prune-Apple Hot Cereal

1 tablespoon uncooked rolled oats

¾ cup water

1 small apple, peeled, cored, and chopped small

5 dried prunes, chopped

1. To prepare either hot cereal, place all the ingredients in a small saucepan, cover, and bring to a boil. Turn down the heat and simmer gently for about 5 minutes, stirring occasionally to prevent sticking.

CHEF'S TIP: YOU CAN USE SOME BREAST MILK TO THIN OUT THE CEREAL IF NEEDED—YOUR BABY WILL LOVE IT EVEN MORE.

Baby's Pureed Vegetables

Yield: 4 (4-ounce) jars

You can make this recipe with almost any vegetable, using these same instructions.

2 cups filtered water

Pinch of sea salt

1 large zucchini, cut in medium-size pieces

CHEF'S TIP: THE BRAUN IMMERSION BLENDER WITH THE ATTACHED CUP WORKS REALLY WELL FOR BABY FOOD RECIPES.

1. In a small saucepan, bring the water and salt to a boil. Add the zucchini and cook for 3 minutes.

2. Drain the zucchini, reserving a small amount of the cooking liquid.

3. Using a blender, immersion blender, or food processor, puree the zucchini. Thin with the reserved cooking water if desired.

Fresh Fruit
Kabob

Shredded coconut or
   granola (raw, page 163,
   or regular, page 33),
   for rolling
Bananas, cut into
   bite-size pieces
Apples, peeled, cored, and
   cut into bite-size pieces
Seedless green grapes
Seedless red grapes
Pineapple chunks
Melon, seeded and cubed
Wooden skewers,
   1 per person

Dipping Sauce
Yield: 1¼ cups
8 ounces plain soy yogurt
½ teaspoon ground
   cinnamon
1½ teaspoons vanilla
   extract
1 tablespoon maple syrup

1. Skewer the fruits of choice onto the skewers.

2. In a food processor, blend together the dipping sauce ingredients until smooth.

3. Pour the dip onto a plate. Spread the coconut onto another plate.

4. Hold the kabob on each end and roll it in the dip, then into the coconut, and serve.

Seed Sprinkle

Makes 1 cup

This is a perfect balance of omega oils, calcium, protein, and zinc.

¼ cup hempseeds

¼ cup sunflower seeds

¼ cup pumpkin seeds, roasted

¼ cup sesame seeds

1. In a coffee or spice grinder, grind each kind of seed separately into a fine meal, and then transfer to a medium-size bowl.

2. Mix well and store in an airtight container.

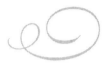

TO SERVE: SPRINKLE OVER OATMEAL, YOGURT, PASTA, OR ANYTHING THAT WILL BENEFIT FROM A NUTTY PUNCH.

Fruity Ladybug Snack

Serves 2

We all know kids love ladybugs.

They will love this tasty snack just as much!

Red apple

Seedless grapes

Peanut butter

O-shaped cereal

Raisins

1. Wash the apple, core it, and slice it in half. Do not peel.

2. Place the apple halves, peel side up, on a plate. Dab a small amount of peanut butter onto the raisins and stick as many as desired onto the apple half to make ladybug spots.

3. Slice a large grape in half lengthwise, and place one of the halves on the stem end of each apple half, to make a head. Slice three smaller grapes in half lengthwise and arrange them around each of the apple halves to make the feet.

4. Dab a bit of peanut butter onto two pieces of O-shaped cereal and stick them on each head, to make eyes.

5. Serve with extra peanut butter for dipping.

CHEF'S TIP: FOR YOUNGER CHILDREN, SLICE THE APPLE INTO MANAGEABLE PORTIONS BEFORE SERVING.

Super Power Fruit Shake

Serves 1

Just the thing to power your little superhero!

1½ cups soy milk, rice
    milk, or apple juice
1 small banana, sliced
¼ cup strawberries or
    blueberries
1 teaspoon flaxseed oil
1 teaspoon spirulina

1. Process all the ingredients together in a blender until smooth.

**CHEF'S TIP: FEEL FREE TO
SUBSTITUTE YOUR FAVORITE FRUIT.**

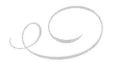

Toddler's Crunchy
Salad Mix

Serves 2

1 beet, trimmed, scrubbed,
    and grated
1 apple, peeled, cored,
    and grated
1 carrot, trimmed
    and grated
¾ cup thinly sliced
    green cabbage
2 teaspoons extra-virgin
    olive oil
Juice of ½ lemon
1 teaspoon rice syrup
    or agave syrup
3 tablespoons sunflower
    seeds
½ cup dried cranberries

1. In a medium-size bowl, combine the beet, apple, carrot, and cabbage.

2. In a small bowl, whisk together the oil, lemon juice, and rice syrup. Pour over the salad and toss to mix.

3. Scatter the sunflower seeds and cranberries over the top and serve.

Trail Mix

Hungry for a snack? This one goes anywhere with you.

Granola (raw, page 163,
or regular, page 33)

Nuts and seeds of choice

O-shaped cereal

Dried fruit of choice

1. Mix all the ingredients together and store in an airtight container. Serve often.

Play Clay

Yield: 1 cup nontoxic clay

1 cup unbleached
all-purpose flour

½ teaspoon salt

2 tablespoons vegetable oil

2 tablespoons cream
of tartar

1 cup water

Coloring

Turmeric (yellow)

Spirulina (green)

Beet juice (red)

1. In a medium-size saucepan, cook the flour, salt, oil, cream of tartar, and water over medium heat. Stir constantly until the mixture is stiff.

2. Let cool and knead out the lumps, while kneading in the food coloring, adding more as required.

Store in an airtight container.

CHEF'S TIP: STORE-BOUGHT NATURAL FOOD
COLORING IS ALSO FINE FOR THIS RECIPE.

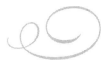

Acknowledgments

Our first thank-you goes to our parents for giving us life. You've always inspired us to be better people and instilled a positive work ethic as well as true integrity. Thank you for seeing us through the challenging adolescent years and helping us to be more passionate human beings.

And thank you to our brothers and sisters for their support.

Gratitude also goes to:

Ginger, for being such a good vegan angel and making the future of the world a beautiful reality.

Our beloved husbands, James Doherty and Jason Silverio, for all the love, for supporting our dream, and for allowing us to be a brighter light to shine for the rest of the world. We love you so much and could never have done it without you.

Judith Weber for her invaluable support, wisdom, enthusiasm, and expertise. This book would not be what it is without her guidance.

Matthew Lore, Renée Sedliar, Renee Caputo, and everyone at Da Capo Lifelong Books, for believing in the book and giving it new life.

Gail's Aunt Evelyn and Uncle Sy for their constant support and inspiration. Lacey's Nana for being an artistic cook and making food fun. Lacey's Grand Mary for making deliciously memorable chocolate cake, cookies, and caramel corn, and Grandpa Ray for loving the sweets.

Elise, our schoolmate and friend, for all her heartfelt work and deep love of all animals.

Hiranth Jaya Singh for help with the food picture styling.

Kit Libenschek for helping us get the first edition of the book together. Without her this book would not have been possible.

Fran Waldmann for the beautiful design of the first edition of the book.

Chef Eric Tucker for his innovative style at San Francisco's Millennium restaurant—you elevated vegan cuisine.

Chef Laura Dardi, a dedicated and fabulous pastry chef and friend who helped us in the formative stages of the restaurant and makes truly delicious cakes and food.

Everyone who supported Down to Earth:

Gabrielle, Regina, Louis, Alexandria, Pat, Eli, Ben, Meghan, Ryan, Taj, Kenny, and Adam for their passion, enthusiasm, and daily inspiration. Jose Gracias for doing such a wonderful job making the kitchen run smoothly and being with us through everything.

Our dedicated recipe testers Sabrina, Stacy, Taj, Wendy, Bruce, Rosanne, Tami, Claire, and Michelle for spending many hours testing and tasting. Trinity for helping us document and refine so many recipes.

Doctor Tommy for turning so many people on to our food and helping us turn the lights on.

Natalie, so much love for hand-carving our gorgeous sign, and Azara for loving food at such a young age.

All the Tiffanys that have worked at Down to Earth, with special thanks to Tiffany Romeo; Tiffany Betts; Kevin, our weekend warrior; Kate; and Wendy Hollander.

Aunt Eva and Uncle Ron for the beautiful paintings and support. Aunt Abby for her enthusiasm.

Cheri Jiosne, André Cholmondeley, Claudia Ansorge, and Ansorge Unlimited for unwavering support.

Cindy, Clayton, Chris, Debbie, architect Steven Michael Peterson, and everyone at Metrovation.

Resources

In this section we give you some sources for most of the ingredients in our recipes, as well as other interesting natural ingredients.

We have also included some of the important organizations that help the world and all its living creatures.

VEGAN FOOD AND COOKING UTENSILS

Pangea
Vegan products
1-800-340-1200
www.veganstore.com

Gold Mine Natural Food
Macrobiotic, Adian foods, pantry staples, and hard-to-find grains and beans
1-800-475-3663
www.goldminenaturalfood.com

Omega Nutrition
Organic oils
1-800-661-3529
www.omegaflo.com

Diamond Organics
Organic produce, groceries, and beautiful gift baskets
1-888-674-2642
www.diamondorganics.com

Maine Coast Sea Vegetables
Domestic and imported sea vegetables and products
1-207-565-2907
www.seaveg.com

Mountain Rose Herbs
Organic herbs and spices
1-415-472-1750
www.wholespice.com

EatRaw.com
Online resource for raw foods and products
1-866-4342-8729
www.eatraw.com

Nature's First Food Online Store
Raw food ingredients and lifestyle products
1-800-205-2350
www.raw-food.com

Equal Exchange
Fair-trade organic gourmet coffee, tea, and chocolate
1-774-776-7400
www.equalexchange.com

Eden Natural Foods
Macrobiotic, natural, and Asian groceries
1-888-424-3336
www.edenfoods.com

Discount Juicers
Juicers, dehydrators, blenders, and water distillers
www.discountjuicers.com

VEGAN SUPPORT

Vegan Outreach
Why Vegan is great vegan information
211 Indian Drive
Pittsburgh, PA 15238
1-412-968-0268
www.veganoutreach.org

The Sierra Club
www.sierraclub.org

The Green Party
www.greenparty.org

The Organic Pages
Guide to the national organic guidelines and standards
www.theorganicpages.com

PETA
People for the ethical treatment of animals
www.peta.org

Farm Sanctuary
Organization for the protection of farm animals
www.farmsanctuary.org

READING MATERIALS

Diet for a New America
by John Robbins
H. J. Kramer, 1998
An informative book on the impact the consumption of animal products has on our lives and on the Earth. A life-changing read. Also on video.

Fast Food Nation
by Eric Schlosser
HarperPerennial, 2002
An exposé and history of fast food.

Food and Healing
by Annemarie Colbin
Ballantine Books, 1986
An informative and practical book on our personal and cultural relationships to food and healing.

The Safe Shoppers Bible
by David Steinman
John Wiley & Sons, 1995
A consumer guide to nontoxic household products, cosmetics, and food.

A Consumer Dictionary of Food Additives
by Ruth Winter
Three Rivers Press, 2004
Easy-to-understand descriptions of more than twelve thousand harmful or desirable ingredients found in food products.

The Book of Whole Meals
by Annemarie Colbin
Ballantine Books, 1985
A look at creating balanced whole meals with philosophy and recipes.

Index